MANIC MINDS

MANIC MINDS

Mania's Mad History and Its Neuro-Future

LISA M. HERMSEN

RUTGERS UNIVERSITY PRESS

NEW BRUNSWICK, NEW JERSEY, AND LONDON

Library of Congress Cataloging-in-Publication Data

Hermsen, Lisa M., 1968–

Manic minds : mania's mad history and its neuro-future / Lisa M. Hermsen.
        p. ; cm.
    Includes bibliographical references and index.
    ISBN 978-0-8135-5157-9 (hardcover : alk. paper) — ISBN 978-0-8135-5158-6
(pbk. : alk. paper)   1. Manic-depressive illness—History.   2. Neuropsychiatry—
History.   I. Title.
    [DNLM: 1. Bipolar Disorder—history.   2. Bipolar Disorder—etiology.   3. Bipolar
Disorder—therapy.   4. Neuropsychiatry—methods.   5. Psychiatry—history.
WM 207]
    RC516.H47   2011
    616.89′5—dc22

                                                                                    2011010852

A British Cataloging-in-Publication record for this book is available from the British
Library.

Visit our Web site: http://rutgerspress.rutgers.edu

Manufactured in the United States of America

For my family, for sharing their very real special powers

CONTENTS

List of Figures   ix
Preface and Acknowledgments   xi

Introduction: Mania's Mad History and
Its Neuro-Future   1

1   Mania Multiplies with Fury: Textbook Descriptions
    of the Psychopathology   13

2   The Maniac and the Iconography of Reform   37

3   Midwestern Mania: Genetics in the Heartland   64

4   Manic Lives: Mad Memoirs   81

5   Neuropsychiatry, Pharmacology, and Imaging the
    New Mania   98

Epilogue: A Mad, Mad World   117

Notes   123
Bibliography   137
Index   147

LIST OF FIGURES

I.1.   Madness, 1806   3
1.1.   "The Dancing Mania," 1564   17
1.2.   "Esquirol's Patient," circa 1830   22
1.3.   Self-decorated manic patient, 1907   27
2.1.   Dr. Philippe Pinel at the Salpêtrière, 1795   38
2.2.   Hospital for the Insane, Philadelphia, 1841   57
3.1.   Pedigree chart of the C___ family, 1911   70
3.2.   Manic depressus, circa 1922   71
5.1.   "The Brain: the Cerebral Cortex," 1537   106
5.2.   "Head and Brain of Adult Human Head, MRI"   107
5.3.   "Straitjacket," 1838   108
5.4.   Frier Hospital, London, a woman suffering from mania, 1890   109

PREFACE AND
ACKNOWLEDGMENTS

When Larry King interviewed *Terminator* star Linda Hamilton on CNN's *Larry King Live* in 2005, he described her as living "a private hell that drove her to drugs, hallucinations, and violent rages." On the show, he promised, she would reveal "how she escaped bipolar disorder, the horror that torments millions." "Hell," "violence," "rages," "horror," "torment"—words like these would dominate my writing and research for the next five years.

I began writing this book on a tour of Philadelphia, when on the advice of a friend I headed to the archive of the Mütter Museum of the College of Physicians. The archivist there shared with me one of the most valuable pieces of paper I own, the handwritten documentation of a case in which a doctor wrote about a patient who was treated by blistering and bleeding but who nevertheless died of a furious mania. This case is still a valuable possession, a reminder of where this book started, even without my knowing it yet.

As this book developed, I was inspired and supported by a network of institutions in Philadelphia. I must begin my acknowledgments with The Library Company of Philadelphia, one of the oldest institutions in the nation and now a kind of second home to me; a very gracious thank-you to James Green for his hospitality there. The Library Company awarded me a fellowship in the Program in Early American Medicine, Science, and Society, allowing me to work closely with many valuable resources. I thank Connie King for her patience as I returned regularly, requesting asylum report after asylum report (well over a hundred in all). I also thank Charles Rosenberg for amassing such a collection and for donating it to The Library Company. Too, I thank Stacey Peeples at the Philadelphia Hospital for allowing me to invade her space one afternoon and read nearly all the hospital's early admission records.

While Philadelphia provided a nexus for my research, a rich source of texts exists in the city where I live, Rochester, New York, at the Miner Library, whose rare-book collection includes first editions of most major psychiatric textbooks.

Christopher Hoolihan was able to find nearly everything I asked for, and started to intuit what I might want and need. He even translated a few lines of Latin. The book certainly would not have been possible without the regular Tuesday afternoons I spent at the Miner.

As for research assistance, I can't say enough good things about Alison Whalen, president of the local Depression and Bipolar Support Alliance/Parents of Bipolar Children/Youth, who works tirelessly with and for parents and their children. Thank you for allowing me to just listen.

I received much advice while completing the manuscript. I want to thank Deb Blizzard, in particular, for talking with me over coffee, suggesting an approach to the introduction, and pointing me to sources.

I gratefully recognize Rochester Institute of Technology for its support in the form of a very valuable Miller Fellowship and for various travel and research grants. I especially thank the former chair of my department, Richard Santana, for protecting as much of my time as he could and for asking about my progress always.

For beginning the publication process with me as editor at Rutgers University Press and adding her editorial comments to the first two chapters of the book, I thank Doreen Valentine. Her work played a role in developing the remaining chapters. For profoundly improving this manuscript, I gratefully acknowledge Audra Wolf, whose sound editorial advice was sometimes tough but always on the mark. Her encouragement was equally essential. I appreciate her close and timely reading, the several long phone calls, and an invitation to tea. I thank Peter Mickulas, who pushed me to finish the writing, let go of the manuscript, and allow someone else to read it. Thank you to Bryce Schimanski, in particular, for moving the book through the last stages of manuscript preparation. Finally, for close editing of difficult passages, thanks to Bobbe Needham.

When asked why I chose to write this book, I rarely dare to reveal my own experiences with mania. By emerging from this diagnostic silence, however, I am able to tell a story beyond my own limited narrative. There were certainly times during the writing when I had to come to terms with the debilitating effects of a manic episode—the bodily reality of psychic tension, times when linguistic power eluded me. But in the end, I hope to have written with the confidence and credibility of one who possesses a dynamic relationship to mania.

A special group of people has been more than friends: Jess, Amit, Laura, and Tim have lived my manias with me (and entertained backyard tackle bocce with a competitive spirit). I am so very thankful to this group of people. I owe them more than I can express. Friends who invited me to yoga until I finished this book: you rock. I thank Rebecca and Dave for opening their den and inviting us in. To my colleagues who never doubted this book would finally be finished, thank you for believing.

For their advocacy and constant work at helping me live without significant episodes of mania during the course of what was an emotional process, I am grateful to my professional supporters: my psychiatrist, Dr. L—, my psycho-therapist, Dr. C—, and my favorite yoga instructor, Amanda.

My parents visited when I needed to take a break, and they came to see me when I was struggling. They fixed lamps, did laundry, oiled squeaky doors—all while I sat at my desk stuck on a single sentence. They took me on long mean-dering walks through the park because they knew I was scared. My sisters texted and phoned and put my life in perspective. This project has both excited and aggravated me over the last several years, and it was my family particularly who helped me sustain my sanity. Thanks to them all for giving me devoted support—and for being willing to do so twenty-four hours a day.

My husband, Rich, got me into this project by bringing me to The Library Company on our first romantic weekend away together. While he introduced me to the joy of good sushi, he also introduced me to the joy of a good archive. Since my first find that weekend, he has been nothing but encouraging. He had not yet seen the torrent of my moods then, but he does not love me any less now that he has. His truly grand gesture, a move from his home in Buffalo, New York, to our home together in Rochester, likely saved me and the manu-script. Because he always works with me to search for the right words, I am unspeakably thankful.

MANIC MINDS

INTRODUCTION

MANIA'S MAD HISTORY
AND ITS NEURO-FUTURE

Toward the close of the [eighteenth] century, mania still wore its earlier garb.

—Andrew Scull, *Social Order/Mental Disorder*

I showed up for my intake interview on Halloween 2003 as an obvious, almost clichéd, figure of madness. I had been performing a kind of madness in various ways for years with deliberate imprecision. I wasn't actually crazy all the time or everywhere. There was little clarity or rigor—no method to my madness. Nevertheless, I had shown up for this interview wearing my Halloween costume: the black widow with fishnet stockings, shoes with heels meant more for seduction than mourning, a nearly too-short black velvet skirt, a gossamer top, long black silk gloves, a black wedding veil, and a large fake diamond ring. The only clue to the essence of the costume—a tasteful sterling pin in the form of a spider. I met the messy questions about impulsive behaviors, excessive spending or sexual activity, and suicide intention or ideation with extrapolated and rambling attempts to give honest but elusive responses. I explained vehemently that my fantasies were not of suicide, exactly. I did not want to kill my *self*, just my *brain*. I urgently needed to stop it. I described a fantasy more imaginative than any mere suicide attempt, a scene in which I clawed at the skin at the back of my neck until layers of muscle fell to pieces, so that I could grab hold of my spinal cord and wrench the entire system—brain and every connected nerve ending—out of whatever would be left of my body. I left the office diagnosed with a manic disorder and prescribed the pharmaceutical cure, lithium.

I did not recognize myself as a mad woman or a maniac. In fact, I'm told it is best not even to think of myself as bipolar. I have an abnormal neurotransmitter system. To be more precise, I have irregularity in my protein kinase C (PKC) signaling system, increase in my dopamine and noradrenaline neurotransmission, and dysfunction in at least two discrete brain structures (the orbitofrontal and medial frontal cortex). These abnormalities had assembled in my brain and were embodied as a piercing, profoundly strange invisible but pervasive pain. The task of accurately describing my mania is wholly unsatisfying. Neither eccentric memoir nor clinical terminology can provide all that is necessary for a suitable appreciation. My mania is a raging fury and a dysregulated neurotransmission with an enduring (partial) connection to madness at its intersection with a potential neurofuture.

MANIA'S MAD HISTORY

From classical to nineteenth-century psychiatry, "mania" described a general category of insanity and could be used interchangeably with such words as "lunacy" or "insanity" to characterize the agitated, furious, and sometimes rageful insane. But while "madness" and "lunacy" have, for the most part, disappeared from contemporary clinical discourse, "mania" remains in use in the clinical psychiatric vocabulary. To put it mildly, then, in the contemporary diagnosis of mania as mental illness, the maniac has occupied "a wholly unenviable ontological status"[1]—the iconic figure chained in an asylum cell (see figure I.1).

Prominent medical historian German Berrios, however, has argued that no plausible history of mania can be written. He warns against reading the mania of the past through the lens of the present. He has rightfully noted that what might have been named "mania" in the first century bears little relation to the disorder classified today as bipolar and to the defining manic episodes. Berrios has wondered, in fact, whether historical examinations of mania provide more than merely a history of a word.[2]

I argue that the word matters, and that a rhetorical history of mania, no matter how messy, can be written—one that pays close attention to the layers of description that have framed mania from classical Greek medicine onward. Indeed, I show that even twenty-first-century definitions of madness remain steeped in the "pertinent words" of psychiatry's earliest practitioners. In this rhetorical history, semantic content and linguistic translations carry the residue of concepts that have been regularly connected over time. Since Hippocrates, mania has been described as excitement, with fury or anger as the primary distinguishing emotion. The International Neuropsychological Society refers to the Greek etymology of "mania" in its dictionary as "madness, from *mainesthai*, to rage."[3] Even as language has shifted and changed, meanings and concepts converge. My book is important because it illustrates how mania has always persisted as multiple objects, often enacted at the same time.

Aretaeus of Cappadocia (150–200 CE), in *Chronic Diseases*, provides the earliest authoritative description of mania as a condition marked by excess:

> If mania is associated with joy, the patient may laugh, play, dance night and day, and go to the market crowned, as if victor in some contest of skill. If it is

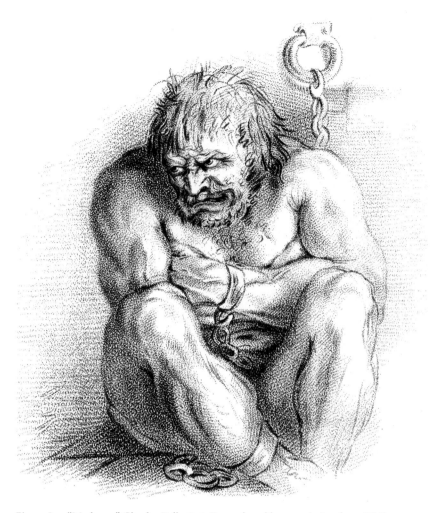

Figure I.1. "Madness," Charles Bell, 1806. Reproduced by permission from Wellcome Library, London.

associated with anger, the patient may tear his clothes, kill his keepers, and lay violent hands upon himself. . . . The ideas the patients have are infinite. Some, if intelligent and educated, believe they are experts in astronomy, philosophy, or poetry, . . . while some uneducated may have strange delusions; ([for example,)] someone would not drink, as fancying himself a brick, and fearing he should be dissolved in the liquid. . . . If the illness gets serious, the patient may become excitable, suspicious, and irritable. . . . His hearing may become sharp but his judgment is slow. Some get noises and buzzing in the ears . . . or may have visual hallucinations. . . . The eyes of the patient may become hollow and may not blink. . . . At the height of the disease, he may have bad dreams and his sexual desires may get uncontrollable. . . . If aroused to anger, he may become wholly mad and run unrestrainedly, roar aloud, flee the haunts of men and go to the wilderness to live by himself.[4]

Aretaeus's maniac informs descriptions of mania from classical to contemporary psychiatry. The sufferer of mania laughs and dances all night, turns grandiose, reverts to delirium and furor, becomes insensitive and dangerous, and finally lives out a life of unreason.

Certainly, meanings of the word "mania" have expanded and multiplied as much as narrowed or differentiated. "Mania" until the nineteenth century described both a general form of madness and a unique variety of madness marked by rage, fury, excitement, delusions, and euphoria. Mania has always existed as madness, and it now exists in our contemporary diagnoses as an episode, a syndrome, a pole on the affective spectrum. When madness is classified as "mania" and is incorporated into twenty-first-century clinical categories of mental illness, madness does not simply disappear. In the twentieth century, the American Psychiatric Association's *Diagnostic and Statistical Manual of Mental Disorders IV (DSM IV)* describes features of a manic episode that resonate with those offered by Aretaeus:

> The expansive quality of the mood is characterized by unceasing and indiscriminate enthusiasm for interpersonal, sexual, or occupational interactions. For example, the person may spontaneously start extensive conversations with strangers in public places. . . . Although elevated mood is the prototypical symptom, the predominant mood disturbance may be irritability, particularly when the person's wishes are thwarted. . . . Inflated self-esteem is typically present, ranging from uncritical self-confidence to marked grandiosity, and may reach delusional proportions. Individuals may give advice on matters about which they have no special knowledge. Despite lack of any personal experience or talent, the individual may embark on writing a novel or composing a symphony or seek publicity for some impractical invention. Grandiose delusions are common. . . . The person may go for days without sleep and not feel tired. . . . Individuals may talk non-stop, sometimes for hours on end. . . . Speech is sometimes characterized by joking, punning, or amusing irrelevancies. . . . Increased sexual drives, fantasies, and behavior are often present. . . . Unusual sexual behavior may include infidelity or indiscriminate sexual encounters with strangers.[5]

According to the *DSM*, for behavior to be considered manic, "the disturbance must be severe enough to cause marked impairment in functioning or to require hospitalization to protect the individual from the negative consequences of actions that result from poor judgment" (American Psychiatric Association 2000). Aretaeus's first-century maniac is a shadowy figure of madness that haunts mania in its twentieth-century classification as mental illness.

In the history of the maniac, perhaps no moment has drawn greater attention than "Le geste de Pinel." In this myth, Philippe Pinel, the heroic symbol of modern moral and rational psychiatry, in 1793 orders the chains removed from the maniacs—the asylum patients—at Bicêtre, a hospital in France. The stories that survive to describe this event, one written by Pinel's son, Scipion Pinel, and the other by his student, J.E.D. Esquirol, describe Pinel poised like a gentle reformer, liberating his patients and inventing a new psychiatry. For some time, Pinel was indeed held up as the symbol for reform, even revolutionary change, in psychiatry. He argued that madness could be treatable and might be curable, provided extensive observations and individual case histories, developed methods of diagnosis and therapy, and divided general insanity into differential categories. The legend of Pinel's "gesture" has been widely circulated and celebrated as a moment of modern achievement, even if most would agree now that the facts do not support a simple or literal interpretation of events.

If Pinel's role in premodern psychiatry did not include the mythic gesture that unchained asylum inmates, he remains a mythic figure nevertheless, for the gesture pointed toward the empirical observation that made possible a scientific classification and a mechanism of treatment that allowed for the curability of some forms of madness. The notable difficulty for Pinel's description of mania, however, is that while Pinel emphasizes curability, he defines mania as unreasonable, violent, and impulsive behavior, and thus both succeeds and fails to transform the image of madness.[6] Pinel's ambiguous place in the history of mania is best symbolized, I would argue, not by the asylum gesture or lack thereof, but by his work of distinction and classification, which "turns out to be the most reactionary, putting the retrograde image of the 'raging maniac' back into circulation."[7]

Michel Foucault offers the most prominent and critical reinterpretation of the history of madness, and of Pinel's mythic gesture. As Foucault notes, the image of a lucid Pinel unchaining the frenzied maniacs who surrounded him carries the weight of legend "at least until today," and underlies the celebrated nineteenth-century asylum psychiatry "which Pinel is credited to have founded."[8] Foucault charges Pinel, with his powers as a medical personage, with the confinement (rather than the release) of the maniac by reducing madness to the status of mental illness. Specifically, for Foucault, madness hollered in the wild until it was silenced by its classification as mental illness, laden in contemporary clinical discourse "with the connotations that are familiar to us today."[9] The experience of madness was once one of animality, free and untamed. Now, modern psychiatry has preserved that animality as immorality, and it is imprisoned in asylums and hospitals. Rather than shaping a history of madness in a linear progression from the treatment of the mad with classical violence to the treatment of the mentally ill by objective human science, Foucault details a rupture in which madness has been excluded from a new medical space. Perhaps if pure madness can be heard at all now, it is only outside the moral discourse of "mental illness," in a place outside the controlling social systems of disease classification.

According to Foucault, madness now sounds only in avant-garde literature, where language breaks free from its representational responsibilities, plays with excess and taboo, and becomes intentionally transgressive. Jean Baudrillard makes the argument that Foucault's *History of Madness* mirrors the history it describes. The text is a work of art that manages a relationship between unreason and reason, a literary masterpiece written with an allegorical, mythical, and legendary language of unreason. The argument Baudrillard and others convincingly make is that Foucault's seductive myth is not a discourse of truth. It is "no truer than any other" and "has no illusions otherwise."[10] I find Foucault's *History of Madness* a wonderful piece of literature as well as a history and a philosophy, a key work in his oeuvre, allowing him to speak the language of madness while leaving mental illness to those of us who would remain imprisoned by insanity. Key concepts from Foucault's work are indispensable for thinking through this version of a history of mania.

For the rest of us, madness may yet elicit desire for a new discourse, one free from confinement. Madness has never been fully exiled from the medical space of psychiatry. It persists in an inexhaustible manic fury. That is, madness has not been, as Foucault would have it, mastered by mental illness. Throughout this book, I use "madness" to mean a wild and untamed madness, a likeness of the maniac in the woods. This general madness continues in the language of contemporary classifications of mania. Aretaeus's "madness" is not the American Psychiatric Association's "mania." But these are not mutually exclusive; rather, they are robustly coordinated. When I refer to "mania," I am always aware that it has been wrapped up in a general category of madness. It has also been separated out into a specific classification of madness. Now, "mania" adheres both to general madness and to its special classification of mental illness—it is never just one or the other. Sometimes mania is almost interchangeable with madness, and at other times it becomes mental illness. Madness clings to mania, and mania is still very much in the making as a medical object. The challenge is to look for how mania comes to be made as madness, as mental illness, or both. The challenge, in part, will be to look at how we use the concepts when we talk about them. Finally, however, the question is not what mania is—mad or medical—because neither works to describe what mania does or how it acts.

And so this book tells a rhetorical history of mania, mindful first of the classical Aristotelian "rhetoric" and the loosely translated definition: "to discover all the available means of persuasion." An Aristotelian rhetoric is also epistemic—a means to discover what can be known about a subject, given a particular exigency, a complex relation of persons, objects, and events. This rhetorical history begins with texts and then follows those texts through multiple and layered discursive practices. It begins with material texts—asylum reports, memoirs, published studies—and follows these as they circulate in the locations that make use of them. The book is a rhetorical history in its assumption: the rhetoric of madness and mental illness has participated in the historical enactment of mania. The argument throughout the book is that only examining linguistic performances, as well as persons, events, and objects, can make a history of mania possible.

The rhetorical history I advance throughout the chapters borrows Ian Hacking's suggestion that we can study "words in their sites" and "the sentences in which the word is actually used" and with what authority, in what settings, and with what consequences.[11] For Hacking, worthwhile research involves tracing objects and their ontologies—asking what is there, what makes it possible for an object to come to be, and how it interacts with the ways we name it. Tracing objects in this way makes them visible, but always *in potentia*. In this case, tracing mania through words, sentences, and sites makes mania visible as it is made possible and is performed. In this rhetorical history, mania is an acting, living, and moving object. This agenda leads to a fundamental, urgent question: Is it possible to create new types of sentences by which new kinds of mania might be made possible?

Regarding the study of medicine in particular, Annemarie Mol has written an ethnography of disease, treating atherosclerosis as an object with multiple ontologies: *The Body Multiple*.[12] By treating diseases as objects with multiple ontologies, Mol is making two important points. First, she argues that we ought to think more about how we talk about bodies and diseases—that illnesses ought to be thought of as real things that can be pulled and shaped in many ways and practiced in various locations. Second, she emphasizes that by referring to "multiple" objects, she does not intend to say that the same illness is represented differently but that the same illness has multiple realties. She argues that what we think of a single object—here, the object "mania"—may in fact be "more than one." How, she asks, does this distinction matter? Mol poses questions similar to Hacking's and argues for following an illness as it comes to be, as it is performed in its many sites. What does it matter, for example, if we treat mania as if it coexists in multiple realities under a single name? Again, the presumption is that by treating mania as multiple, or "more than one," it might be possible to trace the ways in which mania is real and then interfere to enact some realities in different—and it is hoped, better—ways.

Following this rhetorical approach, tracing words in sites and following mania as it multiplies, *Manic Minds* rejects two potential narratives. First, I reject the progressive history of psychiatry that presumes that mania evolved as a psychiatric classification from its affiliation with general madness to a cyclic relationship with melancholy in manic depression and now bipolar disorder. This narrative risks making mania oversymbolic in the history of psychiatry from classical medicine to an enlightened discipline. Second, I avoid the narrative of medicalization as it has come to be used, as a kind of overdetermined discourse about mental illness. Madness may be medicalized, but not singularly.

Not surprisingly, historical attention to mania has remained mainly clinical, the purview of psychiatrists and of disciplinary publications such as the *Journal of Affective Disorders, Confinia Psychiatria, British Journal of Psychiatry*, and *Psychiatric Annals*.[13] These histories describe a progressive understanding of the concept of mania, identify discoveries such as the circularity between mania and a depressed mood, and profile key figures who played a part in creating more precise classifications for mania. Professor of psychiatry David Healy has recently written the most popular of these studies: *Mania: A Short History of Bipolar Disorder*, offering not just a history but a compelling "biography" of the concept of mania and its evolution.[14] These histories, however, tend to treat madness as if it has now passed away.

The grand narrative of *medicalization* has been popularized by Peter Conrad and widely used as a critique of the psychiatric treatment of perceived deviant social behavior. According to Conrad, medicine is one means by which "society secures adherence to social norms; specifically, how it minimizes, eliminates, or normalizes deviant behavior."[15] I argue that the story of mania as mental illness cannot be managed adequately by Conrad's story of medicalization. As long as this is the only available story, too much is left out: somatic sources of suffering, affect and the embodiment of physiological etiology, and the devastating effect on lives of real people who commit so-called deviant acts as the result of their inability to function with a disordered manic mind. Certainly the history of mania is engaged with the social fabrication of mental illness. The story must be told differently, however, because the status of mental illness is more deeply ambiguous than a story of medicalization can tell. Mania coexists with both madness and mental illness, and this coordination is rarely as fully stabilized as Conrad and other critics would have it.

Because I am not telling a progressive historical narrative or using a contemporary theoretical narrative, I need to describe the ways this book will move forward. The caveat is that no narrative will be able to tell everything there is to tell about the history or the rhetoric of "mania." I have chosen to sketch those spaces that deal most complexly with mania in the making, those in which it is best captured and its coordination with madness and mental illness is most visible. The narrative does not flow from madness to mental illness. It does not travel in only one direction. Rather it turns back and goes forward alternatively at any moment in time. It works as a map, accumulated layers, and coordinated sites.[16] This approach holds the most promise for identifying spaces in which to intervene and deploy a different rhetoric that might bring mania into another kind of being.

I avoid extreme ways of talking about illness: there is no space in which to imagine illness as thoroughly constructed through social control, nor is it possible to treat illness as completely physical, a result of diseased brain function. I am fortunate to have several models from which to borrow and steal vocabularies and different approaches to thinking about the culture of psychiatry and

INTRODUCTION   9

the language of disorder. Emily Martin's book, *Bipolar Expeditions*, deserves special mention.[17] Using the language of performativity, multiplicity, and doubleness, Martin explores the different ways people adapt to the diagnosis of manic depression. She repeatedly demonstrates how people living under the diagnosis cross back and forth across the ambiguous line between rationality and irrationality, and by the end argues that the line is in motion. Although Martin's approach is ethnographical and contemporary, and even if some of the analysis leads us in different directions, my historical approach shares some of Martin's theoretical understanding of the multiplicity of manic performance. Jackie Orr's *Panic Diaries*, Jonathan Metzl's *Prozac on the Couch*, and Janet Wirth-Couchan's *Women and Borderline Personality* have also influenced my approach to mania as something unstable and yet deeply entangled with madness in language and culture and brain/bodies.[18] My approach to a history of mania attempts to avoid the "mistake" that Len Browers identifies of assuming that "social categories are incommensurable with physical ones."[19] Because histories of medicine must work with some kind of dynamism between the social dimensions of illness classifications and real or natural elements of the bodily experience, in the following chapters I deal with mania by allowing for a combination of social and physiological etiologies, one that might coordinate and fragment into madness and/or, both/and mental illness.

I also use vocabularies from social studies of science and medicine to describe mania in the making. I will attribute this theft to a variety of authors: Lorraine Daston, John Law, Vickey Singleton, Charis Thompson, and Isabelle Basanger.[20] All these scholars talk of diseases as nouns, as objects that come into being. They describe the emergence of such objects as performances that are choreographed in practices. Mania may become another and stronger object, or it may collapse and pass away. This is why this book is so important. There ought to be a rhetorical future strong enough to disentangle mania from madness, one that will allow us to think and speak about mania without the stigma of mental illness. I want to know whether "raging fury" is a description that will be left behind and if a "better" mania can be found along the way. For example, might it be found in neuropsychiatry: in "dysregulation in the ventral prefrontal cortex"? The following chapters each collect different rhetorical practices, building an argument along the way: first, that the word "mania" has accumulated a connectivity of words to make up sentences that are pertinent to its history; second, that mania has multiplied so that both madness and mental illness are coordinated realities; and third, that as mania will continue to multiply, it will be pushed and pulled in a neurofuture. Living with multiplicity, as Mol would say, will mean living with doubt. But it will also require us to make good choices about what words to use, how to get it right—how to create something better with which to live.

The subject of this book is an engagement with the assertion posed by some scholars that madness has been mastered by mania, which has in turn been mastered by mental illness. The emphasis throughout is on the multiplicity of mania, its coordination with madness, and its elusive relationship to mental illness. While I engage with mania in this book by authoring a kind of manic incidence, this is not an autobiographical endeavor. Indeed, this book is not an unmediated event. But it is rare for any linguistic event to be so. I am an individual who experiences mania and someone who has authored yet one more means through which mania will perform. Certainly my experience has shaped my access to my subject. It has allowed me to claim the authority to explore the multiple ways mania has circulated among texts and the ways it continues to do so, and has thus, I hope, strengthened the scholarly work that has been accomplished here.

The first chapter follows *the words* that appear in the distributed, though highly coordinated, technical definitions of the condition "mania." Here, I examine the practice of mania as it is categorized in the technical discourse of primary texts—treatises, textbooks, and medical dictionaries—from Aretaeus to the 2005 *New Oxford Textbook of Psychiatry*. This important history frames the technical discourse of mania by Emil Kraepelin, who is regarded as the originator for modern enactment of mania. The Kraepelin concept of mania is still considered the origin of the diagnostic criteria used in the *DSM*. My historical analysis concludes with discussion of the various words (e.g., "hypomania" and "cyclomania") used to describe types of "mania" as it is now understood to be a part of an expanding and constricting "bipolar spectrum." The analysis used in this chapter to describe the word "mania"—the connections, disconnections, and coherent or incoherent picture that develop in the medical literature—grounds the narrative in the rest of the book.

The second chapter focuses on nineteenth-century state asylum reports as they map a coordinated image of "mania." The reports were written primarily by asylum superintendents and contributed to textbook symptomatic descriptions of mania, placing it within a preprofessional context. The collection here includes reports from Pennsylvania, Virginia, New York, and much of the country. All echo the rhetorical structure and strategies of their authors, borrowing, quoting, and repeating information, arguments, and details about asylum care for the insane. They describe the architectural plans for madhouses and recommendations for restraint of maniacs. Each report also describes the asylum's architecture in minute detail. The patients in the asylum are arranged on wings according to the category of their illness, the loudest and most disturbing in the caverns of the asylum. As "restraint" becomes a central theme in this chapter, the word refers not only to chains, muffs, and waistcoats, but also to the methods by which mania was made to fit into a classification system. Not only was physical restraint used to discipline manic patients, but restraint of mania within a class of insanity was used to coordinate madness into categories. The reports were written by well-respected psychiatrists during the late nineteenth century, most of them members of the APA. Yet the collection of documents enact an image of a maniac, a lunatic and madman, chained in the cellar.

The third chapter, "Midwestern Mania: Genetics in the Heartland," examines early assumptions about the relationship of heredity to the making of mania, especially when the more organized language of "family heredity studies" was used to research the origins of manic disorder. The central text is George Winokur's family studies beginning in the 1950s and his "Iowa 500 Study" launched in the early 1970s, just prior to the proposal of the Human Genome Project. Interestingly, researchers like Winokur used Iowa as a place to study heredity in manic-depression because it was a state in which there was a stable population—not very many people moved away, so researchers had access to at least two if not three generations. An overview of the leading work done in Iowa in heredity and genetic linkage shows an impressive attempt to use family of origin to find the genetic links for bipolar disorder.

The University of Iowa took part in a first-of-its-kind collaborative study of genetics and bipolar disorder, which applied one of the largest and most complex research designs in genetic research to detect the multiple possible contributing genes for bipolar disorder. Bipolar disorder was among the first of the major mental illnesses to be studied by genetic linking, researchers suspecting strong genetic disposition. As a participant in this study, I have a unique perspective of its textual layers.

In chapter four I describe a group of memoirs written by those suffering from mania. It acknowledges that no manic individual will manage to produce the same mania—but argues nevertheless that the performances will be associated and can be bundled. The chapter assembles memoirs written by men and women who perform and feel mania in their brains, and too often, in their limbs. This chapter works cautiously, knotting a story about how patients experience madness in the form of mental illness. The memoirs I have selected have not received the kind of attention that popular celebrity memoirs have generated.

The final chapter, "Imagined Mania," gathers the activities of the neural network—the actors that cooperate in the elaboration of the brain—into texts, maps, math, scans, and images. Here, I identify the philosophic questions posed by those who are concerned with the threat of possible new "posthuman" determinist futures posed by neuropsychiatry, and who thus argue for a "new" psychiatry. I avoid making the assumption, common to much of the critical literature, that neuro is dangerous; rather I express an attempt to live with, rather than against, the neurological: pharmaceutical companies and biochemistry, brain scan technologies and neurotransmitters. Because brain scans now seem to carry the promise of neuropsychiatry, the chapter focus will move to PET, SPECT, CTI, MRI, and fMRI, which are used to study regional processes of the brain, and thus develop better maps of the human mind. I note the way technologies are designed and selected to enact mania as a multiple object.

I end this book with a postscript as a participant in psychiatry's mad history, and therefore *not* one of "the lucky few who have the luxury of fearing" a neuropsychopharmacological future.[21] This is a brief admission of advocacy for more research into childhood and adolescent bipolar diagnoses. This controversial subject and its appearance (or disappearance) from the *DSM V* will follow the suggestion presented in the book—that we ask more deliberately how brains and disorders are brought into being, how these are multiply performed, and how we will decide to enact one performance rather than another. That is, rather than ask, What is? we might now ask, How might it still be or have been otherwise?

MANIA ON THE MAKE

Mania is likely no different from other psychiatric disorders in its stability or instability. Most (if not all) objects come into being in multiple ways with multiple realities. Mania has been aligned with psychosis, and it too, has a rhetorical history that could be told. For a time in the nineteenth century, psychosis was listed as a symptom of several types of madness, including mania. Sufferers of mania exhibited symptoms of grandiosity, leading to delusion or hallucination. By the late nineteenth century, dementia praecox—what we now know as schizophrenia—was separated from manic depression. The two illnesses have emerged as the two principal disorders of modern psychiatry. Mania and schizophrenia have sometimes coexisted, overlapping as multiple objects, and have at other times dispersed, excluding one another. The two illnesses shared the symptom of psychosis, debated as "schizoaffective psychosis" or as a distinction between manic psychosis and schizophrenic psychosis.

Mania is a particularly interesting case. It has passed through centuries of documentation, leaving a fascinating inventory along the way, a wonderful site for tracing its making. Because mania came to be in more than one site across many centuries of labeling, with astonishing patterns of words in sentences and repeated descriptions of the same physical acts, there is a story to be told that has yet to make its way into a thick history that is mindful of society, texts, and bodies. *Manic Mind* traces this rich and undervalued rhetorical history by examining medical textbooks and asylum reports, genetic studies, and memoirs. It also reflects on the potential in neuropsychiatry of imaging technologies and pharmaceutical treatments. Mania is still very much an object in the making. It will continue to perform multiply. This is a story about how and where madness is performed, mania is crafted into practice, and mental illness is implicated in social, cultural and political ways.

CHAPTER 1

MANIA MULTIPLIES
WITH FURY

TEXTBOOK DESCRIPTIONS
OF THE PSYCHOPATHOLOGY

At the period of her admission into the hospital Salpêtrière, Mad'e A . . .
has numerous hallucinations, utters abusive and threatening language, and
deals blows upon all around her. The patient breaks everything within her
reach, tears her clothing, goes naked, rolls upon the ground, sings, dances,
vociferates, and rejects the aliments that are offered her.

—Etienne Esquirol, *Mental Maladies*

French psychiatrist Etienne Esquirol (1772–1840), once known as "the crown prince of reformed psychiatry," is still the figure credited in the history of psychiatry with inventing the first modern classification of psychiatric disorders.[1] Esquirol emphasized the importance of observation in case reports, like the observation of Mademoiselle in the chapter epigraph, to refine diagnostic categories. As Esquirol observes this patient upon her admission into Salpêtrière, he observes: "The emaciation, the swarthy hue of the skin, the contraction of the muscles of the countenance, the knit brow, the commissures of the lips convulsively raised, the eyes sunken, often injected and haggard, and the animated, although doubtful look, give to the physiognomy of this maniac, a character which perfectly expresses the disorder and exaltation of her ideas and affections." During the night "she indulges in cries and songs." She passes the months of December, January, and February in the "same state of delirium and excitement," but come July, she is discharged, as there are manifestations of reason and all the functions are reestablished.[2]

Esquirol's *Mental Maladies: A Treatise on Insanity*, published in English in 1845, is said to have transformed classical notions of mania by distinguishing it from general madness. In this book, Esquirol emphasizes an important and enduring distinction between intellectual, emotional, and volitional disorders, a classification system that marks what is described as an unprecedented bridge, an epistemic event: Esquirol's classification of mania as an emotional disorder culminated in contemporary understandings of mania as a mood or affective disorder.

The argument in this chapter, however, is that if Esquirol's concept of mania is to be understood as a bridge, it was a bridge that transported deep-rooted notions of madness to current clinical diagnostic criteria for mania. That is, although the underlying classification system may have changed radically, the symptomatic descriptions of the disorder used for purposes of diagnosis did not. Esquirol's case note—however we understand its bridging work—is thus a convenient starting point for assembling textbook treatments of mania.

Textbooks of psychiatry reveal the ways in which mania and madness have been intertwined, from their origins in classical Greek medicine through nineteenth-century etiologies to their contemporary imaginings in neuropsychiatry. As textbooks have traveled from one site to another, they have been read, studied, and perhaps sometimes modeled. The importance of textbook circulations should be estimated as one piece of a larger movement to organize and systematize the activities of a profession with a specialized knowledge. Of the many important practices that hang together to create mania, one essential practice is the classification of new and emerging technical knowledge, and the circulatory attempt to create consensus within still-porous disciplinary boundaries.

As textbook psychiatry circulated among pre-professional practitioners, transporting classification systems to nineteenth-century specialists, a transition is supposed to have occurred: mania, a vague phenomenon of deviant behavior, was supposed to have been differentiated within classifications of general madness and attached to a distinct variety of disorder. Textbooks constructing more precise classification systems, emerging after the nineteenth century, should demonstrate the growth of a new medical psychiatry. Indeed, classification systems have emerged, and mania has been included among the classification categories, though not always differentiated from its origins as vague deviant behavior.

Textbooks are one among multiple sites in which communities of psychiatric practice harness heterogeneity into simplicity, classifying and categorizing disorders as discrete entities with descriptive symptom clusters and disease courses. This does not mean, however, that textbooks simply provide interpretations of mania, representing different perspectives of different physicians at different moments in time. As textbooks become institutionalized, some texts and certain authors are studied and cited by peers and students, passed down through generations, prized and archived. Mania gains closer or weaker ties to madness as these textbooks regularize their construction.[3] The emphasis in this chapter is on how the coordination between textual practice proceeds, how manic appearances have been passed on by a network of texts, and how these inform later texts. As more and more textbooks come together, classical and contemporary descriptions converge, mixing together in our twenty-first-century diagnosis. Throughout, the figure of the maniac continues to enact furious, mischievous, violent, whimsical, ridiculous, excitable, passionate, sexual, noisy, and foolish performances.

This description of the maniac represents the most enduring pattern in descriptions of mania—appearing in the Greek texts and arriving nearly intact in contemporary form. Madness and mania coexist. This does not mean that we ought to read contemporary meanings into classical descriptions. Nevertheless, mania came into being bearing some resemblance to the madness of its history. The juxtaposition of texts traces madness embedded in mania, remaining in psychiatric classification as a mental illness, less as a banished idea than as a performance in action.

This chapter is organized to highlight how the description of mania comes about as it is embedded in the layering of text upon text. It begins with Hippocrates and classical descriptions of mania, followed by multiplying manifestations through the nineteenth century. The chapter examines Emil Kraepelin's *Manic Depressive Insanity and Paranoia* and *Compendium der Psychiatrie*, the sixth edition of which is considered the source for our primary guide to contemporary U.S. psychiatry, the *Diagnostic and Statistical Manual of Mental Disorders*.[4] A brief interlude introduces mania as treated in Freudian psychoanalysis. This is followed by an overview of the rebirth of interest in mania—and the current controversy and confusion over diagnostic criteria for mania along a softer bipolar spectrum. Although the chapter does not emphasize a linear movement from general insanity to discrete disease entity, or offer a complete overview of professional practices from theoretical nosology to clinical diagnostic criteria—or of a coherent medical model for professional psychiatric practice—it does offer a map or a list that reveals the various enactments of mania through the relationships of textual symptoms.[5]

Enactment One

Hippocrates (460–337 BCE) was the first to systematically describe mania. Charles Goshen quotes Hippocrates, who described "states" of euphoria and depression: "griefs, passionate outbursts, strong desires, fears, shame, pain, pleasure, and passion."[6] A classic Hippocratic meaning of "mania"—a reactive state of rage, anger, or excitement—remains salient. Aretaeus of Cappadocia (150 CE) is perhaps the most cited figure in reviews of literature in the history of mania. Speaking specifically about mania, he wrote that in serious forms of the illness, hearing may become sharp and patients may hear noises or buzzing in the ears, some may have visual hallucinations, and some may have bad dreams and uncontrollable sexual desires. According to Aretaeus, mania may lead to full derangement: the sufferer "may become wholly mad and run unrestrainedly, roar aloud, flee the haunts of men and go to the wilderness to live by himself."[7] In Galen's (CE 131–201) humoural explanation of mania, the condition continues to be understood as excited or raving forms of madness. Caelius Aurelianus in fifth-century Rome described mania manifesting in merriment and then anger. Sometimes, there is fear or dread of things quite harmless. Other manifestations may include prophetic power, confusion, and memory loss. Victims think themselves orators, actors, and gods. There is continual wakefulness and unnatural strength.[8]

It is curious that if the earliest concepts of insanity are so general, so temporal, and so ontological as to render mania "opaque,"[9] the symptom descriptions from before 1800 read remarkably like those since 1800. This assertion is not to suggest that mania has been enacted always and everywhere with the same meaning or that it has progressed linearly through time. Indeed, psychiatry did not exist as a disciplined way of knowing for Greek physicians. Nevertheless, care for the insane is evident in the writings. And a theory for insanity is articulated quite clearly: an excess of black bile, concocted in the blood and stored in the spleen, was theorized as instrumental in madness. But grappling with the theoretical causality alone does not lead to a clear understanding of why our current diagnostic criteria for, symptom description of, and disease category of mania seem unable to escape its vague deviant madness. The pre-1800 textbook language, regardless of its timeliness or theoretical obscurity, remains eminently accessible to our contemporary medical model.

Mania in the Middle Ages is best characterized by epidemic mental illness, the "strange delusion" known as the St. John or St. Vitus dance (1300–1500 CE). This mania was enacted by the performance of a wild dance in which victims appeared possessed, "screaming and foaming with fury."[10] While participants may have thought their wild movements were therapeutic and would bring relief from the saints, others believed the "dancing mania" was caused by demonic attacks or tarantula bites. Observers noted that "peasants left their plows, mechanics their workshops, house-wives their domestic duties, to join the wild revels," and so cities became the scenes of "the most ruinous disorder."[11] The diseased gathered as a swarm of dancers accompanied by musicians (see figure 1.1), traveling the streets from day through night. Dancing mania was a condition of excitement, delirious raving, and wild rage.

Physicians in the early sixteenth century who had started to observe the phenomenon as an object of medical research stressed that causes could be located in the human frame rather than in either demonic or saintly interpositions. Physicians recorded attacks in which victims tore their clothes; laughed involuntarily; howled, screamed, and jumped; and sought all pleasurable experiences. The disease, established as a mental disorder, was later described as excitement of the nerves and derangement of the abdominal plexus. Paracelsus (1493–1541 CE) speculated that mania entered the head after appearing just below the

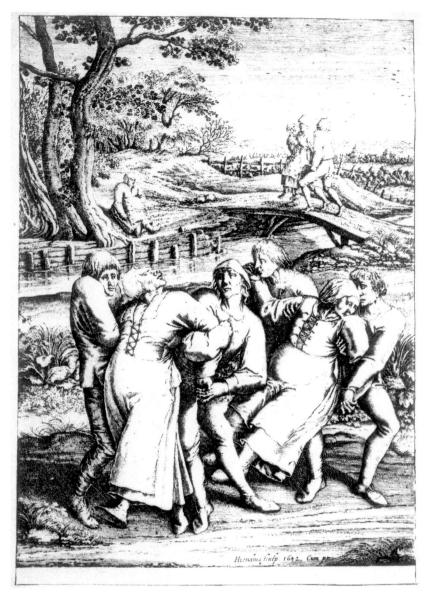

Figure 1.1. "The Dancing Mania," Pieter Bruegel the Elder, 1564. *Reproduced by permission from Wellcome Library, London.*

diaphragm and above the intestines; once the disease enters the head, the symptoms include "frantic behavior, unreasonableness, constant restlessness and mischievousness."[12]

Mania of the Middle Ages is iconic madness. Visualizations of demonic possession or ecstatic corruption remain, even now, lasting presentations of the madman. By the end of the Middle Ages, the visual figure of mania had been well established in medical texts, providing a symbol for identifying the four psy-chopathologies: mania, melancholy, epilepsy, and frenzy. The maniacal figure in visual representations is bound with chains, half-clothed, and contorted—head askew, mouth gaping, and limbs flailing. When the maniac is pictured with others, all in frenzy, the representation of "dancing mania" emerges, as does the dance of the fools. No doubt the "dancing mania" refers to none of the mental functions to which we refer in this century, yet it has both a complex past and a complex present. Its performances have withered but have yet to scatter entirely. The story of St. Vitus's dance cannot all too simply be pushed aside; although the story does not reflect current concepts of mania, these do cohere. The words that describe mania converge to form a partial connection—descriptions begin to overlap and add up. And the iconography of insanity recurs so artfully that the maniac from the Middle Ages onward is ever present—contorted, fierce, ecstatic.

Accounts of mania that advanced from the Middle Ages are strikingly similar to those that came before. Though neither saintly rapture nor demonic posses-sion were as prominent as explanations for mania, eminent medical practition-ers like Felix Platter (1536–1614 CE), whose work was reprinted and read into and beyond the eighteenth century, continued to observe and depict mania as cases of raging frenzy. In his *Histories and Observations upon Most Diseases* (1664), Platter offers portraits of these victims: "Sometimes they are authors of relatively modest words and deeds which are not accompanied by raving but more fre-quently, changed into rage, they express their mental impulse in a wild expres-sion and in word and deed." They exclaim, swear, and behave like animals. They are violent, pull at their hair and clothes, and attack bystanders, trying to bite, scratch, or strangle them. Some go to great lengths to seek sexual satisfaction, inviting the basest of beings to have intercourse. Platter defines both mania and insanity in the same terms: false judgment; eloquent or raving expression; impulsive rage; inappropriate, even animalistic, violent, and self-destructive behavior; and sexual desire.[13]

After the Middle Ages, humoural theories locating mania in the spleen or reli-gious theories blaming the excess of black bile on demons and devils continued to carry authority. However, newer theories of psychopathologies placed mania instead in the nervous system and the brain, and in the blood and heart. In this scheme, emotions were located in the blood, higher intellectual functions in the brain, and the soul in the corpus callosum, an account of madness attributed to Thomas Willis (1621–1675 CE). It is no surprise that Willis, working in the anatomy and pathology of the brain, is credited with inventing a "neurologie," or science of the brain.

Willis, too, describes mania as madness with fury; he differentiates it from melancholia in three ways: "First that their Phantasies or Imaginations are perpetually bullied with a storm of impetuous thoughts, for that night and day they are muttering to themselves various things, or declare them by crying out, or by bawling out loud. Secondly, that their notions or conceptions are either incongruous, or represented to them under false or erroneous image. Thirdly, to their delirium is most often joined audaciousness and fury."[14] Willis also observes that madmen are exceptionally strong, able to break walls and doors, chains and cords. They are almost never tired and almost always furious.

The defining distinction Willis makes between mania and melancholy, the presence of fury, is not original or unusual. In fact, a quick review of the texts thus far reveals "fury" as a distinguishing feature of mania and madness, although Willis and his precursors also define mania by imagined fantasies or false judgments with loud mutterings and cries. Yet despite the proposed psychic causality, they all mention the maniac's fury as the primary symptom for diagnosis. For many, this fury manifests in tirelessness and strength enough to break restraints, including chains.

Hermann Boerhaave (1668–1738 CE), considered one of the most important physicians in Europe, credited Aretaeus, Hippocrates, Galen, and other ancient physicians when he offered his own description of mania as raving madness. When he lectured "Of the Maniacal or Roving Madness," he established a system of diagnostic classification that identified melancholy and mania as two of the most serious disorders. The victim of mania exhibits violent passions, attempting to destroy whatever is displeasing and to procure all that is pleasing. In anger, maniacal persons rage even more furiously, tearing their clothes and clamoring stupidly. Boerhaave depicts the maniac's ravings as distemper, with "an immense degree of strength in the muscles, incredible wakefulness, a wonderful sufferance of hot and cold, with dreadful fantasies, and gesticulations like wolves, dogs, &c."[15] William Cullen (1710–1790 CE), who invented the term "neuroses," cites Boerhaave when presenting his theory of mania in his *First Lines of the Practice of Physic* (1784), in which mania is distinguished by "a hurry of mind, in pursuing any thing like a train of thought, and in running from one train to another." Maniacal persons suffering from false judgments will break out into "violent anger and furious violence against every person near them, and upon every thing that stands in the way of their impetuous will." The disease will also be attended by "a resistance to the powers of sleep" and "that incoherent and absurd speech we call raving."[16]

The definition of mania that begins to emerge in the layering of textbooks and an association of authors is one dominated by the language of fury and rage. Willis, Boerhaave, and Cullen were not alone in turning to the study of the brain. Neither were they alone in carrying forward the raging fury of madness in descriptions of mania. Mention of extraordinary strength, resistance to sleep, erroneous judgment and fantasies, violence, self-destructive behavior, ravings and clamorings appear throughout, along with hurried mind and train of thought.

Clergyman William Pargeter (1760–1810 CE), who advocated for more benevolent care of those suffering maniacal disorders, attempted to qualify the characterization of mania as furious raving. In *Observations on Maniacal Disorders* (1792), he provides a description of mania in which he suggests that fury should be left out of the characteristic symptoms, as maniacs are at different times peaceful and furious. Pargeter does, however, attend to the elements of furious mania: those who suffer "become restless—more loquacious—haughty and supercilious in their demeanor—are suspicious—fickle—captious and inquisitive about trifles—have a furious aspect—redness of the eyes—a quick sense of hearing—are irritable, particularly at meals—they entertain an inveterate aversion to particular persons. . . . They will holler—swear—pray—sing—cry—laugh, and talk lasciviously, almost in the same instant. They have a high degree of salacity—a prodigious degree of strength—a total disregard for cleanliness—are malicious and mischievous, attempting their own lives, or of those about them."[17]

Even eighteenth-century textbooks demonstrate how mania and madness hang together, stay involved, rather than exclude one another. During the era of a more enlightened approach to the science of psychiatry, a shift might have rid madness of mania. If it had, we might find it now difficult to recognize the old madness in the newly conceived disorder. In place of the old descriptions of madness and mania, which would have withered away, distinct language might differentiate madness from new concepts and new descriptions of mania. However, no such radical shift occurred. Madness continued to exhibit partial, though quite intelligible, connections to its history with mania. Pre-nineteenth-century madness as an affirmed *state of existence* (referring to a disordered mind/body in general) passes into mania, now understood as a *state of mind* (referring to a specific kind of disorder). Nevertheless, even with new approaches to causality and classification, the older descriptions of madness appear to remain durable in descriptions of mania, even as it is supposed to evolve as a distinct disorder. Inherited theoretical classification systems for madness (phrensy, melancholia, mania, dementia) and descriptive categories based on empirical observation have always constructed mania as violent fury and agitation.

In the nineteenth century, Philippe Pinel (1745–1826 CE) was among the first practitioners to establish a method for close observation of the insane in order to classify discrete disease entities. Pinel's classification identified "Mania, without Delirium" as a specific disease entity, describing it in familiar language: "I was not a little surprised to find many maniacs who at no period gave evidence of any lesion of the understanding, but who were under the dominion of instinctive and abstract fury, as if the active faculties alone sustained the injury." This perversion of the active faculties was marked by fury, with a blind propensity to acts of violence: "they were under the dominion of a most ungovernable fury, and of a thirst equally ungovernable for deeds of blood."[18] Even Esquirol's (1772–1840 CE) work, which coincided almost exactly in the history of psychiatry with its pre-professional stage, describes the manic with familiar elements: "All at once he fails to recognize surrounding objects, and losing his own identity, lives only a chaotic existence. His disordered and menacing discourses betray the disturbance of his reason. His actions are mischievous; and he desires to overthrow and destroy everything. He is at war with everybody; and hates all that he was formerly accustomed to love."[19]

Esquirol also provides less dramatic descriptions and more clinical symptomology: "In mania, the multiplicity, rapidity, and incoherence of ideas, together with the defect in the power of attention, exalt the passions of the maniac, occasion errors of judgment, corrupt his desires, and impel him to determinations more or less strange, unusual or violent." Esquirol described a syndrome characterized by major abnormalities of affection, including exhalted states, furious rages, inattention, impulsivity, rapid speech and thought, euphoric behaviors, and artistic but incoherent language. He writes that the patient is "led away unceasingly by impressions constantly renewed, he cannot fix his attention upon external objects, which produce an impression too vivid, and succeed too rapidly," or that the patient "associates the ideas most unlike; forms images most whimsical; holds the conversations most strange; and gives himself up to the commission of acts the most ridiculous." He speculated that it was language that disclosed the disturbance in the mind of the maniac. Often, when the maniac speaks, he reveals a brilliance of expression with ingenious ideas. But he can also be incoherent and confused, repeating words or phrases, in rapid and abrupt speech and in variable tones of voice. Esquirol continues with more observations of this kind: "This class of patients fly the light, and have a horror of certain colors. They suffer from a humming sound, and a tingling in the ears . . . and the slightest noise disturbs them."[20]

Esquirol, who originated a supposedly modern clinical system of classification for madness, not only reinvigorates classical descriptions of physical, observable symptoms, but also provides illustrations, an iconography of madness, to accompany specific cases to document insane expression. Esquirol's illustration of mania (see figure 1.2) uses traditional markings: disheveled hair, wild facial features, and bodily disquiet constrained by a straight waistcoat. His descriptions use conventional imagery of "the maniac," who "becomes furious during the night, and utters frightful howls."[21]

Esquirol's classification of mental disorders represents a radical shift from care and treatment of the insane to modern clinical psychiatry. But his depictions of mania carry not only the raging fury of classical madness, but also allusions to its devilish possession and its animalism, as patients are said to become particularly disturbed, acting in mischievous and destructive ways, howling in the night. Radical changes in traditional categories of symptoms, new methods for observing and illustrating symptoms, and new theoretical explanations for insanity were manipulated in practice to sustain the all-too-commonplace objective of associating mania with madness. What might be taken as a new narrowing of the category "mania" and as individuation of insane patients

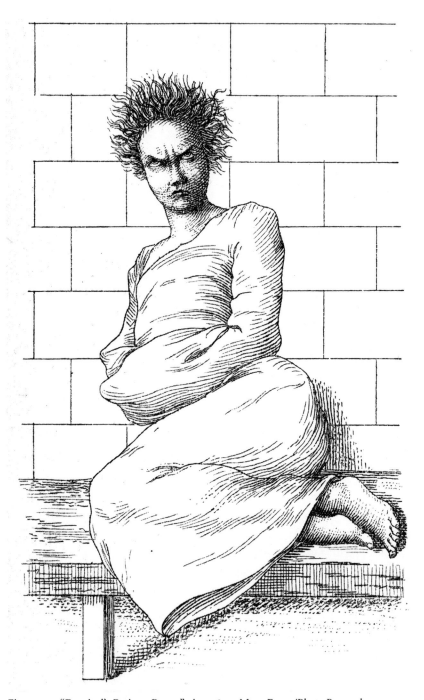

Figure 1.2. "Esquirol's Patient, Part 1," circa 1830. *Mary Evans/Photo Researchers.*

might also be mistaken for classic descriptions of rage and familiar illustrations of categorical madness.

Mania is brought into being here as both a distinctive disease and a general category, without tension between the two. References to and incorporation of Greek definitions of mania and "raving madness" indicate that mania and madness are intermingling, coexistent without confrontation. In some sense, the two depend upon one another. Mania and madness are allowed their ontologies— each realized without excluding the other. At any moment, mania or madness will be sustained or will fall away. And it could have been otherwise. It was never predetermined that madness would progress within the language of mania. It was not a necessary consequence of classification that mania and madness mingle within the frame of raving and fantastic frenzies.

Among the first generation described in the history of psychiatry as a professional psychiatrist, Jean Pierre Falret (1794–1890 CE), a student of Esquirol, provides one of the first introductions of what is clearly recognizable as a rudimentary description of bipolar affective disorder. In "Memoir on Circular Insanity," Falret describes mania late in its cycle: "it is at this point that, if the patients are left to themselves, they turn over their furniture, change apartments, dig up their garden, become mischievous, malicious, and play all sorts of tricks, make plans which they impulsively carry out, compose and write prose and verse; and this prodigious activity, flowing forth in all directions, is present at night as well as during the daytime." Falret's seminal essay documents the complete cycle of circular insanity as a disease entity, and describes the progression of the manic episode as the condition rapidly worsens: "the profusion of ideas is prodigious, the feelings are exalted, great affection is expressed for people toward whom the patient had previously felt indifferent, and hatred flares against those persons who had before been loved the most." While the patient feels "exceptionally robust" and his senses acquire "considerable acuity," he will end up in anxious depression, agitation, or turmoil.[22] As descriptions of mania were limited by tighter boundaries and stricter classifications, its link to general madness ought to have fallen away. And yet, clinical syndromes, as described, converge in words layered with symptoms of classical madness: "exaltation," "mischievous," and "impulsive." A history of the trajectory of mania, linking words in coordination and association, layers and assemblages, tells of inclusion rather than exclusion. Psychiatry's "madness" may seem fragile in the newer classification systems, but it is there. Moreover, classification systems, as noted, are fluid, dynamic, and plastic enough to accommodate multiplicity, and so madness and mania blend.

One of the most popular textbooks from the second half of the nineteenth century, John Charles Bucknill and Daniel H. Tuke's *Manual of Psychological Medicine* (1858), still characterizes mania in "its primary sense" as "that of Raving Madness." In the discussions of mania, Bucknill and Tuke quote from a Dr. Prichard: "the term Raving Madness may be used with propriety as an

English synonym for Mania." The authors make the point that fury is not identical with mania. Nevertheless, they note that by their own observations, maniacs are more susceptible to fury:

> No one will deny that the man who is in a passion, has his feelings rather than his reason disturbed in the first instance; yet when thus aroused, how confused is his language, how distorted is his judgement! He hurries from one unfinished sentence to begin another; his ideas flow too quickly to allow of their sufficiently rapid expression in language. But although Mania in many instances, is a prolonged anger, it may, likewise, be altogether pleasureable in its manifestations, presenting a condition of exhilaration and uncontrollable excitement, in which the patient is rather mad with joy than anger. It is, however, not the less emotional in character, and it is so far a state of irritability, that a very slight amount of opposition would be followed by a display of angry passion.[23]

In the classification of mania, raging fury is symptomatic of the disorder in its fullest development. Due in part to Bucknill and Tuke's text, the old concept of mania as general madness was reportedly placed in a more distinct classification. And yet, while Bucknill and Tuke had placed great importance on devising a classification system, they found some difficulty maintaining the concept of "acute mania" as an independent disease, given the diversity of its symptoms: "Mania may pass, as we have said, into Melancholia; and if these two conditions alternate, it assumes the unfavorable form of circular insanity. . . . Or again, the patient may lapse into Dementia. . . . Indeed, Chronic Mania when advanced is so little distinguishable from Dementia, that the mental condition which one physician would call the former, another would designate as the latter."[24]

The drama of radical change may provide an inspirational and perhaps even influential narrative for the twentieth-century practice of psychiatry as a disciplined medical endeavor; however, the drive for a progressive narrative of mania as something dissimilar emerging from general madness must be tempered by the even more impressive iteration and reiteration of symptoms in the language of textbook descriptions. By the end of the nineteenth century, the practices of textbook classification had built a rhetorical network that connected mania to the madness of its classificatory precursors. A discursive coherence, a bond among definitions and descriptions of mania, can be traced within this circulation of textbooks. In practice, even after the nineteenth century, a demarcation between mania and madness is not secure. It is fuzzy. In this list of textbook descriptions, mania maintains linkages to madness.

Enactment Two

At the end of the nineteenth century, psychiatric classification systems multiplied chaotically and were adopted arbitrarily, with only a hint of systematic consensus. Early twentieth-century psychiatry emerged just outside the medical sciences, simulating a medical model that would mark it with the same science-driven capacity as other medicines, but without reliable and verifiable methods for the diagnosis of differential disorders. Emil Kraepelin's (1856–1926) *Commendium der Psychiatrie*, in its 1899 sixth edition, is considered a historic document, still the basis for the American Psychiatric Association's *Diagnostic and Statistical Manual of Mental Disorders* (DSM), a primary guide for psychiatric diagnosis.[25] Kraepelin's *Clinical Psychiatry* laid the foundations for manic-depressive disorder or what we recognize now as bipolar disorder.[26]

When Kraepelin addressed mania explicitly in *Manic Depressive Insanity and Paranoia*, he began with what he described as extraordinary distractibility of attention: "The patients gradually lose the capacity for the choice and arrangement of impressions; each striking sense-stimulus obtrudes itself on them with a certain force, so they usually attend to it at once." Kraepelin notes that the mood is mostly exalted in mania. In this lively excitement, mania has the "peculiar colouring of unrestrained merriment." In his observation of patients, he notes their expression of such merriment in banter, laughter, jest, and song. When it acquires the stamp of foolishness, however, merriment can lead to conspicuous behavior, especially sexual excitability, he notes.[27]

As mania becomes more severe, impulsive activities also become more intense, Kraepelin records: "The patient sings, chatters, dances, romps about, does gymnastics, beats time, claps his hands, scolds, threatens, and makes a disturbance, throws everything down on the floor, undresses, decorates himself in a wonderful way, screams and screeches, laughs or cries ungovernably, makes faces, assumes theatrical attitudes, recites with wild passionate gestures" (27). The excitement that accompanies the disease may set free certain powers, namely, artistic activity and linguistic expression. Or the excitement may heighten and develop into flights of ideas and pressured speech. The patient talks, screams, bellows, howls, whistles, makes odd noises, threatens, whines, preaches with obscenity in senseless words or syllables, and collapses into unrestrained laughter. Hallucinations are a frequent manifestation, and auditory hallucinations often occur—the patient hears murmuring, whispering, a roaring, crackling, the toll of bells, gnashing of teeth, buzzing of spirits, tones of cursing, weeping, or groaning (9).

Kraepelin remained agnostic about etiology, believing only that the cause of mental disturbance was something unknown and thus unhelpful in developing a definitive classification system. His disease classes, like those proposed by others before him, were based on symptomology. In his textbook, Kraepelin offers distractibility, flight of ideas, impulsivity, and pressured speech as symptoms. Manic-depressive insanity is, he writes, marked in part by "distractibility," exemplified by patients who "lose the ability to select and elaborate their impressions, because each striking sensory stimulus forces itself upon them so strongly that it absorbs their entire attention." A "disturbance of thought" is described in similar terms: "a definite line of thought cannot be followed out; ideas pass abruptly from one subject to another." This lack of train of thought gives rise to what Kraepelin calls a "flight of ideas" (31). In the manic phase, expression of emotion is unrestrained, and there is a tendency to tell jokes and burst into boisterous laughter. Too, in the manic state, there is visible a "pressure to activity," or volition to impulsive behavior (26). The pressure to activity may be present in excessive business, or rise to unrestrained activity without fatigue. There may also be present a pressure of speech in which speech patterns, slang, rhymes, and sound associations are produced as these come to mind. In this state: "patients prattle away and shout at the top of their voices" (32–33).

Kraepelin describes a pure manic state: "the patient cannot sit still or lie for long, jumps out of bed, runs about . . . mounts on tables and benches . . . takes off his clothes, squirts in the bath, bites, spits." And "not rarely are they dirty, pass their motions under them and smear things with their evacuations" (65). He presents a manic patient (see figure 1.3) who has ornamented himself with torn strips of clothing. This photographic representation works within an already established collection of images linked to the manifestation of madness. Here, the expression, particularly the eyes, and the restrained hands and torn clothing map onto the iconic trope of insanity.

Kraepelin describes patients who are "mischievous," who experience delusions in which they claim to have supernatural powers, and who are shameless in seeking sexual excitement. At this point, the descriptions of mania should be familiar. The argument that madness is transported by the descriptions and symptoms of mania should be predictable. What is worth noting are the subtle forms by which the life history of madness is sustained by the textual practices that carry it forward. Madness has its own life history, and it has yet to come to an end.

Indeed the textual influence, from Hippocrates to Kraepelin, is evident in the various editions of the *Diagnostic and Statistical Manual of Mental Disorders*. The first edition, published in 1952, represents a first step in documenting technical knowledge integral to the reproduction of an expert system like psychiatry. It included "manic-depressive reactions" within the psychotic groupings of mental disorders. The first edition of what would later be shorthanded "the Manual" was not a widespread success in coordinating the diagnosis within the profession. When revisions were made to this edition, the word "reactions" was dropped, as was the emphasis on biopsychosocial factors. Diagnoses were separated from unverifiable etiological theories of disorder. The third (1980) and fourth (1996) editions of the *DSM* have been assembled by "neo-Kraepelinian" research groups. Neo-Kraepelin researchers mindfully follow Kraepelin's approach to naturalistic, quantitative, and experimental research methods, avoiding etiological speculation and prejudice, and assuming mental illnesses are "natural disease entities" in need of further clinical verification. When extensive revisions were made to the third edition, the *DSM-III*, in 1980, it was quickly credited with transforming U.S. psychiatry for the twentieth century and

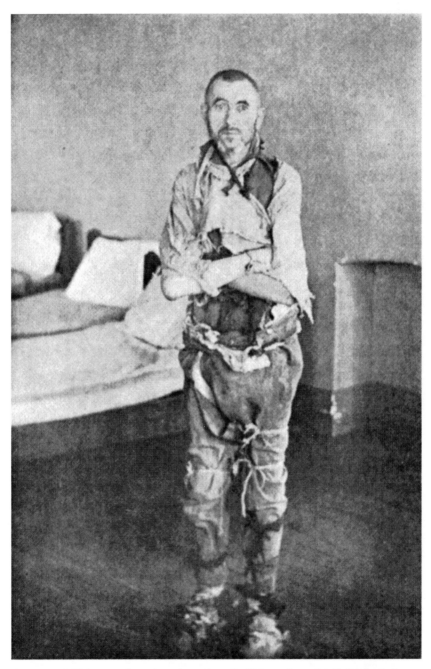

Figure 1.3. Self-decorated manic patient. *From Emil Kraepelin and A. R. Diefendorf,*
Clinical Psychiatry: A Text-Book for Students and Physicians *(1907), in* Lifetime
Editions of Kraepelin in English, *vol. 2 (Bristol: Thoemmes Press, 2002), plate 11.*

beyond.[28] Conditions changed from "neuroses" to "disorders," reflecting the lesser authority of the psychoanalytic community. More importantly, this edition is marked by substantial rethinking of diagnostic criteria. The manual's claim for "reliability" rested on research and on formal, operational criteria to be applied in diagnosis. The third edition included deep structural changes in which disorders were redefined—differentiated, fused, incorporated, or eliminated. This edition replaced the term "manic depression" with the term "bipolar disorder," thus naming the defining feature (mood polarity) of the disorder. The latest *DSM*—the fourth edition, text revision (*DSM-IV-TR*)—arranges subtypes of bipolarity along a continuum or spectrum. The *DSM-IV* carries more influence than ever in the mental health system, from insurance payments to judicial deliberations, affecting the welfare of countless individuals. It has become the most widely used taxonomy, cross-nationally, for both teaching and clinical practice.

The *DSM-III* and the *DSM-IV* are perhaps the most influential actors in medicalizing psychiatry late in the twentieth century. The manual in these later editions has been described as a disembodied mechanism that works as an integral piece of the psychomedico complex, a tool of Foucauldian surveillance that organizes the day-to-day practices of clinical psychiatry. Nevertheless, no edition of the manual claimed diagnostic validity until the 1980 version, which emerged then in the midst of ambivalence as to its reliability and skepticism as to the practice of psychiatry in general. Even in 2007, after the emergence of the revised fourth edition and in anticipation of the next, 2012, edition, the *DSM* has yet to organize expert systems of knowledge—it has been regarded as suspect because of its multiple revisions more than understood as operational based upon the "correctness" of its principles.

Here is a summary of diagnostic criteria for pure mania as indicated in the *DSM-IV-TR*. An "expansive quality of the mood is characterized by unceasing and indiscriminate enthusiasm for interpersonal, sexual, or occupational interactions."[29] Marked grandiosity may reach delusional proportions: "despite lack of any particular experience or talent, the individual may embark on writing a novel or composing a symphony or seek publicity for some impractical invention." Manic speech is characterized by "joking, punning, and amusing irrelevancies." Individuals talk nonstop for hours, may become dramatic and theatrical, loud and clanging, sometimes accompanied by singing. Speech may also become hostile, marked by angry complaints and tirades. Psychomotor agitation is characterized by restless behavior, including pacing, excessive participation in multiple activities, or holding multiple conversations simultaneously. Impulsivity often leads to excessive involvement in pleasurable or high-risk activities, particularly increased sexual behaviors. During this increase in activity, "some individuals write a torrent of letters on many different topics to friends, public figures, or the media." Again, emphasis in the description of a manic episode is on expansive mood, inflated self-esteem, unwarranted optimism, marked grandiosity, and poor judgment. Manic episodes result in severely impaired functioning, delusions, and psychosis, often requiring hospitalization.[30]

The *DSM-IV-TR* remains the primary classification system for mental disorders, and like any other classification system, it has grown out of a history—entangled in cultural, material, and linguistic webs. To fully understand the significance of the *DSM* is to understand it not as a sacred scientific text, but as a circulating object. It is one more text in a gathering of textbooks. It has become sometimes more and sometimes less real, depending on its ability to link otherwise scattered phenomenon, to firm up coherent categories, and to stabilize criteria for inclusion and exclusion. When the *DSM* classification system is more positive, more scientific, and more real, its assemblage of diseases is more real, as well. Thus this description of mania gains reality. But classification systems, though powerful, are almost always messy. As the *DSM* changes in its future editions, it may become more fragile, unable to sustain cooperation among ranks of researchers. The pertinent questions here are not, Is the science sound? or Are the politics suspect? but, How is the classification system—more specifically, how is mania—assembled out of madness? and What effects does it have? That is, what is at stake? It is not surprising that the "psy-sciences" have had difficulty solidifying mania within their practices as an object in the world.[31]

The description of manic symptoms that informs twentieth-century diagnostic criteria differs so little from the descriptions in every century prior that mania is not only intelligible, it is tangible. Perhaps the underlying causality, differential diagnosis and classification, disease course, and treatment and prognosis have undergone a transition of magnitude beyond the scope of this chapter, but the symptom cluster that has been operationalized as criteria integral to qualify mania as a disorder has been transported from text to text to text without transformation. By now the descriptions are more or less shocking—because of their too-close proximity to this century and the popularity of the *DSM-IV-TR* for diagnosis more than for the repetitive immediacy.

The textbooks layered here may modify the meaning of the word "mania" as they carry definitions forward. But meanings multiply rather than go extinct. If we cannot or will not get at the root of the patterns, we will not find the traceable associations that have left mania with its madness, in its elusive and unenviable status. The manic condition may have arrived in the twentieth century in modified, mediated, or distorted theoretical form, but for the most part, the textbooks have served as mere intermediaries, linking traceable associations between mad fury and mania and mental illness.

FREUDIAN INTERRUPTION

As revisions were being prepared for the second edition of the *DSM*, a parallel movement—psychoanalysis—had taken hold as the dominant psychiatry.

Editors of the *DSM-II* clearly responded to psychoanalytic philosophy when they replaced the word "reactions" after disorder names with the word "neuroses." Although this change might have seemed minor, it indicated the predominance of a psychoanalytic movement. Between 1952 and 1980, as significant revisions for the *DSM-III* were hotly debated and slowly drafted, psychoanalysis provided an alternative explanation for mental illnesses.

In the early twentieth century, soon after the Second World War, Freudian psychoanalysis developed as an international movement, and disorders previously expressed in biological or neurological terms were more likely now to be defined in psychological terms. This moment has been described by historians of psychiatry as "the Freudian Age." Freud redefined etiology and diagnosis in terms of libido theory, attending to hysteria, anxiety, and obsessive neuroses by pointing to problematic familial relationships or individual development as causes of mental illness. Symbolic trauma and unconscious psychosexuality were treated in office-practice psychotherapy.

The "Freudian revolution" of the early twentieth century is typically thought to have radically shifted psychiatry's focus from somatic to psychological models of mental illness. According to Freud, depression was a neurosis and thus a functional disorder, treatable in a psychotherapeutic setting. Mania, however, was a psychosis and an organic disorder. The polarity of a manic-depressive is the polarity between a neurotic and a psychotic mind. In the Freudian interpretation, manifestations of manic behavior are due to a lessening or cessation of the oppression that the superego habitually exercises over the ego. Maniacs are people whose superego temporarily merges with their ego after having strictly ruled it, that is, the super ego and the ego have fused, so that "the person, in a mood of triumph and self-satisfaction, can enjoy the abolition of his inhibitions, ignore his feelings of consideration for others and his own self-reproaches."[32] Freud himself described, fully intact, the manic episode—elation, excitability, flight of thoughts, increased self-esteem, feelings of omnipotence. Even within a Freudian psychoanalytic frame, increased eating, drinking, smoking, and sexual activities characterize the manic condition. Impulsivity leads to more social engagements, money is spent freely, new ventures are undertaken without hesitation, and there is much less regard for convention. Typically, talk is loud, vulgar, or profane. Violent destructiveness is common. The severity of the disease may manifest from mild excitability to frenzy.

The "revolution" that shifted focus from somatic to psychological models of mental illness merely contained the same somatic representations within yet another (though not alternative) description of symptomology. This revolution, however, did reimagine older "polar opposite visions of insanity."[33] Disorders were now divided into commonplace distress and major psychotic disorders. This revolution is mainly responsible for medicalizing—or, more appropriately, pathologizing—social distress.[34] This observation has not escaped scholars of trauma, who note that psychoanalysis did indeed pathologize modern distress—it also pathologized mania by distinguishing neurosis from psychosis. General unwellness was treated as neurosis; the maniac, in its reincarnation, was treated as an uncontrollable psychotic. During what has been called the "crisis in psychiatry," psychoanalysis held out little hope for those severely disordered.

Histories of psychiatry have assumed a more radical shift away from psychiatry to psychoanalysis and back than can be supported. While psychoanalysis may have peaked between 1940 and 1970, psychoanalytic ways of conceptualizing mental disease continue to the present.[35] In fact, while the 1970s are supposed to mark an end to psychoanalysis and a return to biological psychiatry, the canonical textbook, the *Comprehensive Textbook of Psychiatry*, by Alfred M. Freedman, Harold I. Kaplan, and Benjamin J. Sadock, includes in its 1975 second edition not just "remnants" of a prior psychoanalytic regime, but evidence of reliance upon multiple episodic events. For example, the textbook describes mania in Freudian terms of regression (as when sufferers eat their own feces) and as a denial and loss of inhibition (when propriety, convention, and discretion are painfully absent). Layered onto these descriptions, the *Comprehensive Textbook* also offers the hallmark psychiatric definition of affective disorder: elevated, expansive, or irritable mood. And, not surprisingly, these psychological and biological approaches to mania intersect with a symptomology offering the now uncannily familiar description of madness. Coexisting on the same textbook page with regression, inhibition, and elevated mood, the maniac's "excessive good humor is transformed instantly to the most vicious anger" as he demands the center of the stage, punning, teasing, and cracking jokes—"some of them good, some awful, some coarse, some blasphemous."[36]

The *Comprehensive Textbook of Psychiatry* is useful not only for emphasizing the multiplicity of madness and mania throughout the history of psychiatry, but also for anticipating its multiple future. In the century since Kraepelin defined manic-depressive insanity, the concept of mania has expanded in bipolar disorder, emphasizing pure mania, as well as hypomania and mixed manic states along a more fully developed soft continuum. The authors seem to anticipate this research agenda and its implications. When the textbook describes mania as one end of a spectrum, it begins with a somewhat positive representation: "There are some people blessed with unquenchable gaiety and energy. They soon become the center of every group they join. They may sound somewhat superficial, but are nevertheless alert, quickly seize upon a new idea, develop it energetically, and manipulate people and things in the environment to ensure its acceptance. They are the movers and doers of the world."[37]

This representation applies to only less severe manic manifestations— hypomania, a newly classified disorder; the hypomaniac "appear[s] as one of God's anointed."[38] It is in acute and delirious mania that symptoms become more intense: sufferers are incontinent (both running at the mouth and urinating) and hallucinatory. Included here are notions of divine inspiration, animality, and immorality. The textbook, familiarly known as "Kaplan and Sadock's," is important because of its ability to perform a mutual inclusion of practices— Freudian analysis, manic symptoms, and mad spectrums.

ENACTMENT FOUR

As emphasis on a more inclusive continuum has increased in what has been called the "rebirth" of research and bipolar disorder, researchers have grown more uncomfortable with the inherited narrow categorization of mania. A bipolar spectrum with more elasticity has emerged during this rebirth. For example, G. L. Klerman in 1981 proposed a spectrum for mania that included six subtypes within bipolar disorder. D. L. Dunner and colleagues in 2003 introduced the distinction between Bipolar I, with manic episodes, and Bipolar II, with hypomanic episodes. More recently, H. S. Akiskal has argued for an even broader spectrum of diagnostic categories, proposing a "soft bipolar spectrum" to accommodate the nuances of the various subtypes of bipolarity. Akiskal's schema of bipolar subtypes includes:

Bipolar I: full-blown mania
Bipolar I 1/2: depression with protracted hypomania
Bipolar II: depression with hypomanic episodes
Bipolar II 1/2: cyclothymic disorder
Bipolar III: hypomania due to antidepressant drugs
Bipolar III 1/2: hypomania and/or depression associated with substance use
Bipolar IV: depression associated with hyperthymic temperament.[39]

One of the largest concerns with the expanding bipolar spectrum is the distinction of hypomania from mania—a distinction or a spectrum from functional or normal to pathological and impaired. A popular model of the bipolar spectrum distinguishes Bipolar I by the occurrence of a manic episode and characterizes Bipolar II as accompanied by at least one hypomanic episode. In this spectrum, Bipolar I, with manic episodes, is a severe disorder with the potential for psychotic or schizobipolar variants. Bipolar II is less severe, characterized by spontaneous and recurrent hypomania with excitation over one or two days. However, within this spectrum and others, definitions of "hypomania" are open to quite a bit of debate—and controversy. In fact, "there is no generally accepted operational definition for hypomania as a diagnostic parameter."[40]

If mania is defined by full-blown symptoms, hypomania is understood as a less severe manifestation of those same symptoms. Although for mania, symptoms are "complete," for hypomania, they are similar though "low-key." For example, the *DSM-IV-TR* emphasizes that delusions are present in manic episodes, but not in hypomanic episodes. The description of hypomania also emphasizes that, in opposition to mania, the episodes have no psychotic features and do not result in enough impairment to warrant hospitalization. In addition, the symptoms include change in functioning marked by an "increase in efficiency, accomplishments, or creativity." Grandiosity is limited to inflated self-esteem, and there is no flight of ideas. Impulsive activity can be goal directed or risky but is usually organized and "not bizarre." Critics have noted that hypomania might be perceived, based on its description, as an attractive disorder.

Certainly, when hypomania is described as a bipolar disorder with "lesser manic intensity" or "below the mania threshold" or simply "less than mania," this mild mania is also less recognizable as madness. The suggestion has been posed that more patients will be politely diagnosed with "hypomania" as an alternative to the pejorative "mania."[41] Dr. Ronald R. Fieve in 2006 published a self-help book that introduces Bipolar IIB (beneficial) as a condition with "hypomanic advantage." He notes that Bipolar II, when diagnosed and treated, can lead to productive highs, increased energy and enthusiasm, and intensified creativity.[42] Other self-help advocacy offers similar help, for example, *Finding Your Bipolar Muse: How to Master Depressive Droughts and Manic Floods and Access Your Creative Power.*"[43] These books are in line with those written by research psychiatrists Kay Jamison and Nancy Andreasen, who posit a special connection between mental illness and creativity.[44] Lana Castle's *Finding Your Bipolar Muse* is aimed at those who want to manage this connection more effectively—to schedule creative time and run a creative business effectively and with financial success. As does Fieve's text, Castle's book emphasizes not the life-threatening dangers of bipolar disorders, but the advantages of bipolar subtypes associated with less severe mood disorders.

These various descriptions of hypomania highlight the disagreement about the best way to understand mania and its subtypes. Is mania becoming (or will it become) more loosely described as hypomania? Are all affective disorders merging, manifesting along a continuous distribution of moods, without the clean natural boundary between mania or depression and "normality"? Or will mania and hypomania come to be two distinct types of disorders, in which mania either more or less (or simultaneously both) will resemble its former manifestation as madness, or become distinguished as a narrowed disease entity by its more extreme symptoms? The group of bipolar affective disorders is "extremely heterogeneous," and classification is ongoing. Continued use of a narrow bipolar spectrum could result in underdiagnosis or delayed diagnosis. A more inclusive spectrum might account for episodes "beyond classic mania."[45] As the bipolar spectrum extends and blurs, mania either will include hypomania, mixed states, cyclothymia, schizoaffective disorder, and some types of "atypical" psychosis, or it will remain differentially diagnosed with symptoms of madness—or it will fall away and wither into these various fragments.

If the history of mania has been told, in part, as a narrowing of mania from general madness to a discrete disease entity, it is difficult to characterize the twenty-first-century bipolar spectrum disorder, with its inclusion of mood regulation from mania to depression, with or without distinct boundaries.

The new "bipolar spectrum disorder" is still in flux, with mania on a continuum. Somewhere along the margins of the continuum, mania is touched by madness, an old concept now appearing in new vocabularies, marginal but not vanished.

CONCLUSION

For some historians of psychiatry, the history of mania is developmental. In this understanding of mania's history, the concept of mania parted ways with the old madness by transcending a simple enumeration of symptoms and achieving a more distinct classification. There were various evolutionary changes along the developmental path to a contemporary concept of mania. After the eighteenth century, the theoretical classification of symptoms gave way to naturalistic observation and differential diagnostic categories. One important shift was the change in the clinical concept of mania, defining it as an affective disorder as opposed to the intellectual or volitional disorders. The very notion of mania was changing as hypotheses were multiplying, and yet mania persisted as a name for a condition with close associations to madness. These theoretical shifts did little to change mania, insofar as they were not fundamentally incompatible with the all-embracing language of madness. Another related change has been described as one from a contextualized approach (in which mania was linked to onset by certain life events) to a medical model (in which mania was linked to a disease course and brain disorder). In truth, such a history is all too tidy. To be fair, the story is one of twists and turns.

Mania in its current form cannot be and ought not be thought of as differentiated from madness in psychiatry's distant history. Whatever the theoretical underpinnings, whatever the etiology, mania is still dependent on the old system of symptomology. The rhetorical history offered in this chapter does not attempt to sift through the various medical manipulations of mania to discover what classification system, which clinical observations, what set of symptoms, or which diagnostic concepts—or even what disease entity—really depicts mania (or, for that matter, which claims priority).

As neuropsychiatry turns mad symptoms into "regions of interest," it is yet to be determined how "mania" as an object in the new disorder will be handled. Nothing is sure; there is more than one reality; it might always be otherwise. Neuropsychiatry will continue to assemble mania. Will it be possible for us to ask, not whether we have discovered the real mania, but whether we are handling mania in a better, even a good, way? And might we ask, not whether mania is really madness, but what does this link do, and how might we now enact other and better links?

According to Kaplan and Sadock's seventh edition of their *Comprehensive Textbook of Psychiatry*, classic mania has been formulated and operationalized as a "manic episode," as mood disturbance: "elation, euphoria, and jubilation, typically associated with laughing, punning, and gesturing." This jubilant mood is unstable and turns so excessive that patients become irritable and hostile. In this description, the "hallmark" of mania is heightened activity, pressured speech, flight of ideas, impulsive and meddlesome and intrusive behavior. The list of examples of manic behavior includes "preaching or dancing in the street; abuse of long-distance calling; buying new cars, hundreds of records, expensive jewelry, or other unnecessary items; paying the bills of total strangers in bars; giving away furniture; impulsive marriages; engaging in risky business ventures; gambling; and sudden trips."[46] Authors contributing to *The New Oxford Textbook of Psychiatry*, one of the leading textbooks among twenty-first-century students and clinicians, use what is now a very recognizable, even conventional, description of mania as elevated mood, pressured speech, racing thoughts, heightened energy or irritability, and distractibility.[47] As mania worsens, the patient talks more and in a louder voice. There is intrusive behavior, arguments, and attempts to dominate others. The patient clearly believes he or she possesses grandiose abilities, revealed in symptoms such as reckless driving, risky financial investments, or exhibitionist sexual acts. Also included in the textbook description, however, are the associations between mood disorders and regional structural brain abnormalities: the limbic portion of basal ganglia and brainstem structures. The old psy-sciences and the neurosciences have started to convene.

Even before the end of the twentieth century, the contemporary psychiatric gaze had turned to the simulated image of neuroscience, so that the gaze now streams on a much, much smaller scale along the systems of neurotransmitters. New objects will come into being—neurons, metabolites, glutamate, receptor sites, and so on. Neuropsychological research reimagines the heterogeneity of the bipolar spectrum, the cognitive function in episodes of mood disturbance, the distinctions between manifestations of mania in Bipolar I and Bipolar II, and phenomena during periods of euthymia (normal mood state). Textbooks continue to enact mania, not by symptoms alone, but now also in terms of brain mechanisms. Mania is performed throughout these textbooks in images of brains and these "regions of interest"—the prefrontal cortex, the right posterior orbitofrontal cortex, and the left ventromedial prefrontal cortex. As the brain performs certain activities, the performances of manic brains are linked in colorful scans to "trait-related" phenomena—sustained attention, memory, executive function (i.e., inhibitory control), and emotional processing (including behavioral changes and impulse control).

In this hinterland, the concept of mania may have loosely cohered out of the more scattered madness, disentangled from wild webs of spirits, priests, and beasts, into a more restrained object. However, even in this brief moment, as mania and madness are reshuffled and transformed, mania yields layers of mad symptoms. There is no dispute here that psychiatry (like nearly every other realm of society) is prohibitive, regulatory, and reductive. Certainly, there is a psychiatric industry that provides institutional surveillance. The amendment to this criticism is a reminder that psychiatry also can be performative, can be productive, and can multiply. What theories of medicalization leave out is the possibility of this instability. While the classification of mania participates in defining deviant behavior, it has yet to be so fully medicalized as to have contained its deviance. To describe what madness, or mania, or mental illness "are" requires tracing what is bundled together, what holds to what, and to describe the ties between madness and mania and between mania and mental illness in a shifting—perhaps crumbling, but certainly provisional—assemblage. The task of this chapter has been to wrangle "mania" out of the assemblage, from the multiplication of its textbook histories, so that its future alterations, translations, or substitutions might be traced in the next chapters through its practice as described in reports from the asylum, in genetic studies, and in neuropsychiatric research.

CHAPTER 2

THE MANIAC AND THE
ICONOGRAPHY OF REFORM

Experience, however, has happily shown, in the Institution whose practices we are attempting to describe, that much can be done towards the cure and alleviation of insanity, by judicious modes of management, and moral treatment.

—Samuel Tuke, *Description of the Retreat*

Definitions of mania that traveled out of textbooks and into asylum reports in the first years of the nineteenth century created the most famous iconography of the maniac and his "liberation" out of the dungeon and from his chains. Tales of violent maniacs brought to their reason, calmed without resort to violent restraint, provide vivid portrayals of the great unchaining and the coordination of rhetoric in asylum reform. Philippe Pinel in France and Samuel Tuke in England compose strikingly akin accounts: when a potentially violent maniac unexpectedly threatens to attack with a rock or stick, the physician approaches the maniac, not with mechanisms for physical control, but with conviction and reason. The physician commands the maniac with a resolute tone of voice and a calm gaze of the eye. With this expression of determined intent, but without vexation, the physician convinces the maniac to correct his conduct. Pinel details a specific account:

> If a madman suddenly experiences an unexpected attack and arms himself with a log, stick, or a rock, the director—always mindful of his maxim to control the insane without ever permitting they be hurt—would present himself in the most determining and threatening manner but without carrying any kind of weapon, so as to avoid additional vexation. He speaks with a thundering voice and walks closer toward the maniac in order to catch his eye. At the same time the servants converge on him at a given signal, from behind or sideways, each seizing one of the madman's limbs, an arm, a thigh, or a leg.

Thus they carry him to his cell while thwarting his efforts and chain him if he is very dangerous or merely lock him up.[1]

Tuke tells a very similar story:

The maniac retired a few paces and seized a large stone, which he immediately held up, as in the act of throwing at his companion. The superintendent, in no degree ruffled, fixed his eye upon the patient, and in a resolute tone of voice, at the same time advancing, commanded him to lay down the stone. . . . He then submitted to be quietly led to his apartment.[2]

These two separate but like accounts describing the dangerous maniac submitting to the gentle but stern physician bear witness to the humane principles and rhetoric of reform: if the most furious and dangerous raging maniacs could be released from their chains and possibly even cured, the revolutionary ideals of asylum might be realized.

Pinel and Tuke symbolize the myth of asylum reform. The grand story of Pinel's revolutionary gesture—"Le geste de Pinel"—marks the ceremonial moment in which Pinel liberated the mad, ordering iron chains removed from the maniacs at Bicêtre Hospital in Paris.

Pinel's gesture, repeatedly evoked as daring precedent, has been famously celebrated as the starting point for a growing conviction that chains inflicted unnecessary pain and degradation. Although Pinel's more dramatic story has

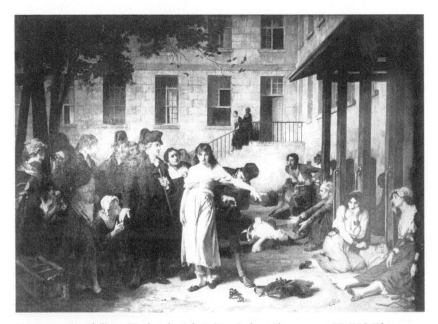

Figure 2.1. Dr. Philippe Pinel at the Salpêtrière, Robert Fleury, 1795. *PR INC./Photo Researchers.*

earned him a crucial place in the history of asylum reform, Tuke's reformations ran parallel to Pinel's and likely developed independently, if not as publicly. Tuke prohibited the use of shackles and unnecessary violence at the Retreat near York in England (a practice established by his grandfather William Tuke in 1796). There he experimented instead with principles for moral treatment, expressly for humane care of the insane. The symbolic stories told by Pinel and Tuke were celebrated by their successors for centuries. The accounts provided by the two men were later printed and distributed, circulating widely in France and England, reprinted and recounted in the United States by asylum superintendents, democratic reformers, and public figures. However, these descriptions of the liberatory gesture and the humane management of the disciplined maniac have been reread by historians who argue that these are mythical ideals—merely legendary in value.[3] Although the myth may not entirely capture the agile performances by which the fantasy of the asylum was built or the cure of the insane guaranteed, it does depict, for the figure of the maniac, different realities—occupying at once the core and the margins of asylum reform. Thus Pinel's gesture, even if mythical and legendary, worked in practice to enact this figure as doubled, made and remade, classified through various kinds of synchronic ambiguity: driven at once by a furious mental disorder and a moral social order, curable if confined early, and chronic once confined to permanent care.

For Michel Foucault, who provided the most influential interpretation of the gesture in his *History of Madness*, the physician's gaze in confrontation with the maniac does not symbolize liberation. Rather the "absolute gaze" evokes the power of confinement, classification, and cure. The gaze confines the madman, not for diagnosis and proper treatment, but as an object of observation. Raging mania becomes visible as a specific class of madness, and this class is made available to the gaze only so that respectable tactics for restraint of all unreason could be discovered. The gaze does not offer up a cure—it establishes the physician's victory in a battle of wills. For Foucault, the asylum had become a battlefield and psychiatry the battle. While Pinel and Tuke may have gestured toward a psychiatry that was to become "medicine of a particular style," this gesture marked only the moment that psychiatry began to remake madness in the new positivist status of mental illness.[4] According to Foucault, the treatment of madness during reform did not progress to the treatment of madness in the modern human sciences. Once the mad were chained by physical restraints and confined to asylums; now the mad are made into objects of scientific observation, their madness pathologized. Foucault's history of madness articulates the cultural structures of power by which madness is determined to be curable and thus determined to be a mental illness.[5]

The history of mania—and the figure of the maniac—is a necessary supplement to Foucault's story, articulating how this particular species of madness has come into being (is still coming to be) as a multiple object, neither mad nor ill, but both mad and ill. The maniac plays a troubled role and acts as an unwitting

figure in the battle between him and his physician within an even newer system
of psychiatry—a network of neurotransmitters, neuroscience, and neuropsychiatry. Even in this history (and perhaps especially so), we cannot escape the
myth of madness liberated or the grand gesture by which the myth has been
passed on. Mania was identified as a "class" of madness, one among four
primary classifications, including melancholia, dementia, and idiocy. Of these,
mania was repeatedly referred to as the *worst* class of insanity, improved very
little by moral treatments. Too, because the maniac exhibited obscene symptoms, he was banished to asylum corridors far away from other patients so that
he would not bother, insult, or badly influence those of higher habits of mind.
The figure of the maniac was enrolled in the double rhetoric of curable and
chronic madness. The myth of the gesture could become the fantasy of reform
realized—if the maniac, the classical figure of madness, could be cured.
However, the gesture remains fantastical—if the maniac, performing the most
violent class of raging madness, remains undisciplined and thus restrained, if not
in chains, in "refractory" asylum wards designed for their more secure, if less
comforting, care. Once the fantasy of reform fades, the maniac became entangled in the rhetoric and reality of asylum custodial care. Mania that improved
could be classified as an acute illness, but mania that did not improve was left to
chronic madness.

U.S. reformers inherited from this mythic fantasy a rhetoric that could support a discourse of cure even for the worst class of madness, acute mania, or the
long-term management of those suffering chronic mania. This rhetoric justified
asylum not only at its core, but at its margins, available outside the asylum to the
nation's public in a "communication culture." By the midnineteenth century,
a revolution in communication (invention of the telegraph, improvements in
print technologies, spread of print periodicals) was arguably "a driving force
in the history of the era."[6] New and controversial ideas in favor of and against
state funding for asylums and private philanthropy for retreats, embedded in
utopian dreams of democratic reform, were publicized, discussed, and dissemi-
nated. Debate about the construction of insane asylums and the implementation
of moral treatment for the raging mad from every class of society appeared in
legislative petitions, spread through pamphlets and newspapers, and made
its way into literary magazines. Reformers wished to further their efforts by
educating citizens about the success of therapeutic treatment for the insane
and calling for acceptance of expanded roles for the asylum in such treatment.
Descriptions of the asylum and its accommodations, its superintendent and
its patients, were accessible to the public in this communication. Everywhere
in these documents, the maniac—more than the melancholic or demented—
appears as a central character in the battle for public opinion. The maniacal
patient suffered the highest form of madness and thus provided the most useful
rhetorical force in asylum narrative. His seclusion in an institutionalized collectivity of madness allowed this figure to become more (rather than less) visible

within the public and political movements both for and against reform. But the maniac never remained sequestered in the province of asylum medicine. The figure eloped from the asylum to create whole communities of raving maniacs performing in popular print, from newspapers to literary magazines to the penny press. The maniac became intertwined with the common culture of asylum reform and a communication revolution, and coproduced as a material and metaphorical body.

ASYLUM REPORTING AND RE-FORMATION

The "asylum era" in the United States has been dated from just after 1750, when the Pennsylvania Hospital first began treating insane patients as a specialized institutional practice under the care of Dr. Benjamin Rush, through the nineteenth century, when insane asylums were constructed for more "enlightened" treatment after the model introduced by Thomas Kirkbride. Throughout the asylum era (1770–1895), the center of care for the insane moved from the home or the general hospital (or almshouse or jail) to specially designed institutions, as the practices of asylum medicine and "moral treatment" came to offer curative promises.

The Pennsylvania Hospital—the first institution in the colonies to provide medical treatment for the insane—admitted insane patients, assuming that with institutional care, such persons might improve and perhaps even be cured. In the worst case, the insane would be protected for the safety of themselves and their families or communities. Although the admission of insane persons to the hospital represented a shift in the treatment of insanity, for the most part only the dangerously insane were actually admitted to the hospital. One request for admission from March 1765 states that the potential patient "is so much disordered in his senses, that it is apprehended he might murder his wife or do harm to some other persons."[7] The hospital also accepted the wandering insane from communities unable to provide appropriate care for the insane person or protect themselves from the disordered lunatic. The following petition describes such a case:

> October 1769
> We the subscribers do hereby certify that _____ single woman is an inhabitant of the said township and she having been for sometime past crazy and out of her right senses and having no friends or relatives to take care of her nor estate or substance to maintain herself, we recommend her as an object to be taken to the Pennsylvania Hospital and we will during her stay there provide for her necessary clothing and receive her again when there unto required and also pay the expenses of her burying if she happens to die while in the hospital. Witness the hands . . . [8]

Treatment for cases of insanity remained mainly that of secure custody in basement cells. When severe cases were placed in hospital care, physicians relied primarily on techniques that would subdue furious behaviors: bloodletting, blistering, and immersion in cold baths.

Between 1751 and 1883, asylums were erected along the Eastern Seaboard from New York to Massachusetts and Virginia, across the Midwest from Ohio to Iowa and Kansas, and throughout the south from Kentucky to Tennessee and Georgia. Almost every state in the union had built (sometimes multiple) public institutions for the insane. In each asylum, a superintendent served as a "medical man" or a chief physician, responsible for treatment of insane patients. Nineteenth-century U.S. asylum keepers professed reform in the treatment of insane persons, insomuch as dreary cells were converted into comfortable, domestic abodes. No longer confined in chains and forgotten in dungeons, the insane were cared for in carefully designed structures with well-lit hallways, airy rooms, and common spaces. The founding thirteen members of the Association of Medical Superintendents of American Institutions for the Insane enacted a vocational philosophy based (in part) on three major principles: prompt commitment, differentiation of classes of patients, and complete recovery for curable cases, with assurance of competent custodial care for chronic cases. As the association grew to more than fifty members at the height of the asylum era, these major principles were choreographed as the basis for shared practice.

Admission records for the Pennsylvania Hospital diagnose patients in fairly rudimentary terms: insanity, lunacy, madness, and melancholy. Asylum reports began to identify more distinct classes of insanity, diagnosing patients as inflicted with mania, monomania (or partial insanity), dementia, melancholia, hypochondriasis, or idiocy. Some reports build more elaborate categories for diagnosis of forms of insanity by differentiating, for example, among varieties of manic insanity: mania; mania of the melancholic, epileptic, homicidal, or suicidal variety. The reports used statistical tables to identify not only the class of insanity but also the number of patients identified as suffering from each class. For example, the 1839 *Annual Report of the Directors of the Ohio Lunatic Asylum* lists the species of insanity and number of patients as:

Mania: 101
" of melancholic form: 17
" epileptic: 12
" homicidal: 4
Moral insanity: 10
Dementia: 10
Idiotism: 3[9]

The asylums were built with the principled ideal that patients in any condition of insanity or from any economic standing could be accepted into the asylum and receive appropriate treatment. While the wealthy might have been expected to pay for their room and board, those of lesser means would have been asked to pay a lesser amount for their care. Even the insane paupers, disagreeable and filthy, were taken in rather than turned out into poorhouses or penitentiaries. The arrangements in the asylum, however, provided more refined and cultivated accommodations for the more refined and cultivated classes. For those who could afford the best housing, there were single rooms with views of the landscape, the portico, and the porch.

As the asylum became the standard of care for the insane, the superintendents believed the architecture of their buildings was especially important for providing a curative environment in which moral treatments could best be carried out. The Kirkbride model asylum, built according to guidelines published in 1851, certainly influenced asylum architecture at the height of this era.[10] The Kirkbride model was a linear plan that arranged short corridors in a V-shape so that every room had an unfettered view of the landscape. Asylums were state-of-the-art institutions with technologically advanced fireproof construction, heating and ventilation systems, and fresh water supplies. They were surrounded by natural landscapes with walkways and flowers, gardens, and even small farms. Although specific architectural plans varied from asylum to asylum and changed over the course of the century, select principles of design persisted as significant influences in the construction of buildings housing the insane.

The guidelines offered by the model of the "purpose-built" asylums emphasized the importance of an architectural plan for successful moral treatment, imitating a kind of domesticated space with ample light, accessible dayrooms, and furnished parlors.[11] There were common rooms with musical instruments and reading materials. These domesticated wards seemed to be the exception, however. Amicable gentlemen and women took advantage of the privileges of moral treatment provided in the best asylum architecture. Those who disturbed the domestic environment, in either the evil of insanity or manner of habits, would be removed to nearly uninhabitable spaces of the asylum (either designed to be fully detached or reserved as a corridor at a distance). The wards for the mad and underclass had to be separated from the others if moral treatment for those who could benefit from it was to succeed. Patients who responded to moral treatment worked in gardens or sewed clothing, and often dined in the great room with the superintendent, almost as a family. Others scrubbed hallways and cells or washed laundry. And many who were not of the higher classes, either of sanity or of society, dined in a common space at a common table. Some maniacs were considered so frenzied as to be unaffected by moral treatments and were provided shelter without advantages of work or of company. The asylums were built to satisfy a hierarchical space that explicitly evoked the "excitable" class in the hierarchy of insane classifications and then coordinated this "obscene" class with the hierarchy of social classifications.

The cure for mania was manipulated within an exceptional tool of control for the preservation of social order, choreographed in the nineteenth century as a revolutionary improvement in the progress toward medical psychiatry. New asylum reform movements were put into practice to enact the cure of mania as possible. Nevertheless, likely neither disciplinary coercion nor the advancements in science adequately account for the asylum in the United States, and neither the oppression of the socially deviant nor medical treatment for the insane are proposed here to explain the systemized techniques and structured practices that materialized as "the asylum." As asylums were invented across the country, efforts at care and cure were haphazard. Early in efforts for reform, arguments for the physician's primacy regarding care and treatment of the insane remained incomplete. Argument for moral treatment as liberation and promise for cure justified no single asylum regime. Indeed, each asylum used different techniques for managing the care of patients—different ways for observing and classifying, different therapeutics, and different asylum architecture. Too, asylums were thought to be tranquil, curative facilities that would succeed in providing comfort and care for the insane without medical intervention. Indeed, the asylum might very well have succeeded through its failure.

Asylum superintendents composed annual reports for the asylum's directing body, providing information regarding the state of the asylum, including the number of patients in residence, the condition of the grounds and building structures, and a detailed account of financial expenditures. The superintendents composed their reports by borrowing, quoting, and repeating information, arguments, and details that echo the rhetorical structure and persuasive strategies of the collective body of their peers. The homogenous quality of the compilation of reports is hardly accidental. The superintendents were well aware that the audience for their reports extended beyond their financiers to the public, who no doubt had heard or read spectacular stories of madmen in institutional confinement, but now heard of equally curious, spectacular claims of madness cured. The authors crafted rhetorical arguments for reform addressed not only to governing and funding bodies, but to the public, whose voyeuristic interest in these institutions was stimulated by allusions in journalistic, literary, and even musical artifacts available throughout the nineteenth century.

The appearance of the seemingly bureaucratic but highly rhetorical asylum reports begs the question of production and consumption, and the consequent power of these texts. Of course, historians who treat the cultures of print—even those arguing that a "reading revolution" marked the nineteenth century—ask important questions about how the changes in technologies of print distribution affected the real practices of readers in a generalized public culture.[12] In the case of asylum reports, it seems their sensational subject, the curiosity of a generalized literate public, and a network of committed reformers would likely have attracted readers interested in the particular subject of insanity and lunacy reform. As the asylum reports circulated among legislatures, information about asylum practice would have also reached a wider public. These seemingly bureaucratic accounts sustained the status of the maniac to demonstrate the necessity of an enlightened asylum reform. Every superintendent assembled and reassembled the highly staged innovations of Pinel and Tuke, who tamed the maniac and reformed madness. The texts were arranged by rhetorical choices, which emerged quite comfortably to compile multiple public, political, and personal motivations into a single simplification: a testimony unanimous among asylum practitioners that the maniac could emerge from the asylum reasonably cured.

The 1813 Philadelphia reprint of Samuel Tuke's *Description of the Retreat, an Institution near York, for Insane Persons of the Society of Friends* made Tuke, as well as Pinel, a model for reform of the treatment of insanity in the United States. The document makes the basic claims for asylum care that would be repeated often in U.S. asylum reports. Moral treatment is distinguished from "terrific" treatments, with chains and corporeal punishments that "fix for life, the misery of a large majority of the melancholics; and drive many of the more irritable maniacs to fury or desperation."[13] An institution practicing moral treatment for persons suffering from insanity can do much "for the cure and alleviation of insanity" (84). Experience at the Retreat demonstrated an advantage to treating persons afflicted with disorders of the mind "in an early stage of the disorder" (38). Furthermore, the classification of patients was considered an essential therapeutic approach. The principle of moral treatment, however, makes an exception in the case of violent mania, when coercion is considered "a necessary evil" (105). The more violent patients who do not possess the capacity for rational enjoyment were to occupy buildings separate from "the superior class, in regard to behavior, and to capacity of rational enjoyment" (65).

The *Appeal to the People of Pennsylvania on the Subject of an Asylum for the Insane Poor* from 1838 refers to the debt owed to Pinel, the "learned French physician," for the American philanthropic spirit. According to the familiar version of the story told again here, Pinel removed the shackles from fifty-three lunatics and an unexpected improvement followed: "The furious madmen, who monthly destroyed hundreds of wooden utensils, renounced their habits of violence; others, who tore their clothes, and rioted in filth and nudity, became clean and decent; tranquility and harmony succeeded to tumult and disorder; and over the whole establishment order and good feeling reigned."[14]

The *First Report of the Physician of the Tennessee Lunatic Asylum: To the Legislature of Tennessee, for 1840 and 1841*, celebrates Pinel similarly for "setting at liberty about fifty furious maniacs, without injurious or dangerous consequences resulting to the other peaceable inmates of the establishment." Perhaps the most embellished account is provided by the physician and the superintendent in an 1842 report to the regents of the Lunatic Asylum of South Carolina: "Who can conceive the feelings of the French philanthropist amid the exciting circumstances that surrounded him!" Pinel, in a revolutionary move, after fruitless applications to the government, "went to the cell of an English Captain who had been in chains forty years and was the terror of all the keepers, struck them off and gave him his liberty." Pinel's experiment was described in this report as "completely successful," as in a few days "fifty-three maniacs were released from their chains." This gesture, says the report, marks "one of the chief glories of our age, that this barbarous system has, to a great measure, been abolished throughout the civilized world, and for it has been substituted, what may be emphatically called, the rational treatment." The report exults: "In the whole record of benevolent emprise, there is not an incident, perhaps that possesses a more thrilling interest and awakens deeper emotion. It dates at the period of the bloodiest of Revolutions, and exhibits in delightful contrast, a spirit of mercy and peace, which appeared, like a Guardian Angel, to stay the general havoc, and point to a brighter and nobler existence."[15]

The U.S. Jacksonian era was one of reform marked by both the achievements and the consequences of a new democracy, following the era of revolution. Not surprisingly, then, asylum reports drew upon Pinel, a French revolution, and lunacy reform to campaign for nationwide struggle on behalf of the insane. Reports make explicit links between this heroic and revolutionary act by Pinel and the equally heroic acts of U.S. physicians and superintendents. In the 1840 *Report of the Superintendent of the Boston Lunatic Hospital and Physician of the Public Institution at South Boston,* Pinel is favorably compared to Americans like Samuel Woodward, who have done so much for the management and for recovery of insane persons that when their work is compared to the "gross errors" of just twenty years ago, the principles appear "almost like revelations."[16] In the young republic, asylum reformers used the mythic though symbolic breaking of chains and liberation of the maniac to highlight the model of democratic freedoms and reasoned republic the asylums intended to adopt.

One of the most famous early U.S. asylums, the Friends Asylum at Frankford, was established outside Philadelphia in 1817 as an American model of the Retreat at York in England. When the Friends Asylum at Frankford hired Thomas Kirkbride as resident physician in 1832, he emphasized in his report of the physicians for that year Tuke's claim that early and proper treatment in the asylum is necessary for cure of insanity. He argues it is "obvious" that the treatment of insanity depends upon the promptness with which it is attended. Here Kirkbride also warns that cure is more likely for those who are confined within the first three months, and that hope for cure steadily diminishes from six to twelve months, and thereafter. Hence, he introduces both possibility for cure and potential for chronic cases.[17]

When Kirkbride in 1841 accepted the position as superintendent of the new Pennsylvania Hospital for the Insane, he outlined his belief: "The general proposition, that truly recent cases of Insanity are commonly very curable, and that chronic ones are only occasionally so, may be considered as fully established and ought to this day be every where understood." Furthermore, only the asylum is prepared to admit cases of insanity, as it is " now well ascertained—that in a large majority of cases, it [insanity] can be managed with success, only among strangers, and generally in Institutions, where extensive provision has been made for a liberal and enlightened treatment of this class of disease.[18] He also repeated the argument that asylum care requires the strict classification of patients. To that end, the Pennsylvania Hospital for the Insane, as it was designed in 1841, used detached structures to house noisy or violent classes of patients. According to Kirkbride, these detached structures were already proving to be a successful addition to the institution, as "some of their inmates, even of the very worst class, have manifested a decided improvement in their habits, from the stricter classification, and more perfect supervision, to which they have been subjected." In fact, proper classification of cases and temporary seclusion had proved so successful that "very little glass has been broken, and many patients have been prevented from tearing their clothes."[19] A later report from the Pennsylvania Asylum, in 1856, refers explicitly to one "case of highly marked mania" that was received "in the early stages" but which developed ultimately "a few weeks afterwards and ended in death." The same report documents cases of acute mania, "one case which was with us but five days." This case was a "very striking example of the highest grade of acute mania, supervening on a chronic form of insanity of some standing."[20]

As Kirkbride outlines the primary tenets of asylum reform, the maniac begins to move around the entangled expectations of asylum practice and across the promise of potential cure. If asylum treatment would be choreographed to cure insanity, this treatment must perform cures or provide care for even the most furious and most dangerous class of insanity: mania. Once enrolled and allied with asylum principles, the maniac could speak to the evidence of those principles. The choreography was performed, in part, by the circulation of texts between "persons who could vouch for one another" and thus turn "a multiplicity of persons into a social arena of authority."[21] Of his own reports and those of others, Thomas Kirkbride remarks: "uniformity of character, and perhaps repetition in details, can hardly be avoided in the reports." Nevertheless, "this is the less to be regretted, as these documents are constantly referred to by different individuals, who expect to derive from them, some knowledge of the capabilities and modes of management of the institution to which they refer."[22] The uniformity with which mania was addressed in conventional asylum rhetoric served to multiply mania, as the arguments for asylum required different messages and additional layers of persuasion. The maniac pathologized as deviant and dangerous coexisted with the maniac who was normalized in descriptions of a diseased organ, a disease that could affect anyone's brain and ought to be treated like a disease of any other organ in the body. In the asylum, the maniac was classified with an ill-defined set of overlapping symptoms and was consistently refashioned. In the asylum reports, mania was altered, manipulated for the public in intersecting conversations of confinement, classification, and cure. The reports translated the mixture of mania into a coordinated madness so that the asylum could be assessed as the best hope for restoring reason to the republic.

ASYLUM RHETORIC AND MANIC DOUBLING

The rhetoric in the asylum superintendents' reports tangled mania in webs of recommended interventions for the mad and therapies for the insane. The reports shaped mania as a particularly difficult class of madness that, if cured, demonstrated the success of asylum reformers, who could provide progressive treatment for the whole of madness. But the reports fragmented mania, with the result that it was coordinated and manipulated in different ways to tell the single story (though with multiple realities) of asylum reform. When mania as violent and dangerous madness came into being as a special class, it also came into being as a class that was handled by removing the maniac from the society of the asylum to be doubly confined in special wards or rooms. When madness was deemed incurable, it was mania that resisted treatment and was deemed chronic. Even as "acute" mania in its violent manifestation could be cured if brought to the asylum with prudent timeliness, "chronic" mania treated with compassionate care rather than restraint provided proof of the success of asylum reform. These dual strategies for enacting mania certainly interfered with one another, even as they were partially connected. Mania emerges as an oscillation between the general and the particular. The maniac represents the class of madness at the matrix of the generic malady. He is a madman. But the maniac was also brought into being as a particular class of madness. He suffers from a uniquely furious, frenzied, and violent pathology. As a generic malady, mania can be cured, but as a class of madness, mania exhibits a kind of chronicity difficult if not impossible to treat.

Mania throughout asylum rhetoric is thus performed doubly, sometimes variably, and perhaps divergently. Interpreting the rhetoric by which those engaged in the practices, treatments, and therapies of mania does not by itself provide a satisfactory picture of how mania and the maniac were handled in asylum practices. The asylum reports no doubt capture many of the elaborate and elusive realities by which people were confined, classified, and otherwise cared for. But the maniac also comes to be in ways that are more than metaphorical—and more than marketable. The maniac comes into being as a material object, a body in an engagement with the inhabited institution of the asylum.

CONFINEMENT

Asylum rhetoric in the superintendent reports made the convincing argument to the community that the asylum alone was suited to treat madness. Quick delivery of the insane to an asylum was the most important act leading to the possibility of recovery. Delay in bringing the mad for asylum treatment might require a longer stay or might result in a chronic condition. The dual ontologies of mania figured in both the necessity of confinement and the probability of deconfinement. Mania remained engaged in a dynamic participation with general madness as violent and dangerous, in need of confinement not only for treatment, but also for the protection of society. But mania was also enrolled as a concrete class of insanity, in need of confinement for treatment rather than merely for the protection of the community. The asylum could offer some consolation for a heightened frenzied distress. The maniac was thus aligned with the dual purpose of confinement. Mania, because it was choreographed as the *most* perverse insanity, required moral and medical treatment within the asylum. But the maniac also participated in general madness, and thus sustained the madman's potential and his capacity for liberation.

Early nineteenth-century reports from the asylums express special concern for "wandering maniacs" and for those who have been wrongly jailed and restrained and who suffer alone without hope of restoration. Like the 1837 *Third Annual Report of the Directors of the Ohio Lunatic Asylum*, the reports recommend care for maniacs within more protected asylum confinement: "The strongest sympathies of human nature should be excited to ward off and mitigate the sufferings of the maniac. He is not a criminal that he should be imprisoned, nor a demon that he should be shunned and abhorred."[23] *The Report of the Commissioners Appointed by the Governor of New Jersey* in 1840 makes the most comprehensive argument for confinement in the asylum by referring to the deplorable lives of maniacs suffering outside an asylum:

> The raving maniac requires to be restrained and confined, but the kind of restraint and confinement which is indispensable to him, cannot be furnished by the penitentiary, nor county jail, nor by any private family. The jail may be security against escape, and manacles and chains may restrain him from doing violence to himself and others, and this is all these can do. They can do nothing towards his restoration. The violence of disease remains unmitigated, and its victim may linger out years of wretchedness in the dungeon, or death may speedily [come] to his relief. An asylum constructed and adapted to the object, we believe can alone furnish the required restraints and remedies.

The arguments for confinement expressed in these reports were arguments for the protection of the maniac from the community or from himself. Once confined, the maniac could improve. The New Jersey report goes on to claim: "The maniac of the most ferocious character, has been here, not cured, but tamed and restored to the comforts and decencies of life."[24]

Many reports promised that a maniac of the most severe annoyance to relatives, friends, and neighbors could be improved by asylum treatment. The 1841 *Report Relative to an Asylum for Lunatics, by the Joint Committee of Council and Assembly, Trenton* describes the "extreme wretchedness and suffering" to which maniacs are exposed and suggests confinement in an asylum as protection from such. The report describes the itinerant insane who are found "chained like criminals to the floors and the walls, from year to year, enduring cold and hunger and solitude and nakedness. They are found in the woods, wandering in the streets from place to place, destitute and friendless—the sport of boys and

wicked men." Here again the maniac is made visible by removing him from the
prisons and the woods and housing him within the comforts and confines of an
asylum. According to this report, however, few insane persons had such comfort: "They are thrown into a cellar or garret, shut out from medical treatment,
to become raving maniacs for life."[25] Descriptions of roving madmen were thus
accompanied by an explicit plea for family and community to admit manic persons to the closest asylum for their best chance of cure—before they lost that
chance altogether.

The reports sometimes included cases of maniacs whose condition
"improved" and thus offered proof of the asylum's restorative, rather than
merely protective, capacities for all who suffered. The following case is presented
by S. B. Woodward in the *Annual Report of the Trustees of the State Lunatic
Hospital at Worcester* in 1835:

> No. 7. Had been confined a violent maniac. Had been caged and chained for
> years. It was concluded to set him free, and see how he would conduct. He fell
> foul of his brother, and killed him with a bludgeon, and, pursuing his sister,
> would probably have done the same to her, had he not been arrested in season
> to prevent it. When caged he was naked and filthy, but now dresses neatly:
> is clean and civil: mingles freely with sixteen other persons, and, though quite
> insane, is to us perfectly harmless.[26]

The case is presented as evidence that even the most violent and dangerous
maniacs can be soothed by confinement in a well-regulated asylum. Similarly,
the *Report of the Superintendent of the Lunatic Asylum of South Carolina* from
1842 boasts: "To see a furious incurable maniac, soothed and quieted, and
reduced to willing subordination, the long-lost peace restored to his agitated
bosom, made industrious and useful, is indeed a spectacle to make glad the heart
of the philanthropist, and which can be witnessed in every well-regulated institution."[27] The *Twenty-Fifth Annual Report of the Officers of the Vermont Asylum
for the Insane* distributed in 1861 confirms these observations: "If the patient be
suddenly attacked with a violent form of mania, or becomes dangerous, and
the friends have not the means of restraining him, he will generally be taken
to an Asylum where the usual facilities and appliances for his recovery can be
available, and he will usually be restored."[28] It is the treatment in addition to the
confinement that offers even maniacs the possibility for improvement and even
recovery.

The doctrine calling for early confinement would be repeated often, frequently with warnings about the danger of deferring treatment. In most cases the
dangerous insane are linked to the deferment of treatment, when the danger
arises that they might become a threat to the community. An important distinction is made in 1863 in the *Twenty-Seventh Annual Report of the Officers of the
Vermont Asylum for the Insane* between those who are violent and thus placed in
an asylum where they can do no harm and the quiet insane who suffer delusions

in secret. Both are dangerous—though the quiet insane may not be confined quickly enough for treatment to be effective. According to the *Report of the Officers of the Iowa Hospital for the Insane* from the year 1866, the hospital continues to "afford asylum to a large number of persons afflicted with insanity" "who would be troublesome or dangerous when at home or at large." Of these afflicted persons, however, there are many for whom improvement is not likely, because they had not been sent to the hospital more promptly.[29]

Asylum rhetoric from the early years of reform through the height of the "age of reform" argued for the confinement of the maniacal insane for safety and for cure. In 1880 *A Report of the Board of Managers, for the State of New York* makes this observation explicitly—and notes a progressive reform from custodial superintendents to "medical" superintendents. According to the report, "the first problem that suggested itself in regard to the management of the insane, was doubtless the protection of sane members of society against the dangerous excesses of such of the Insane as were excitable, furious, or maniacal." The report also describes a second sphere of duty, one connected to medical science and much more dedicated to "remedies" than to confinements.[30]

The various authors of these many reports were aware that they were entering a public debate, and they coordinated a rhetoric that described the figure of a dangerous, violent, raving, and frenzied maniac suffering from general madness as an object to be confined so as to be safe from danger. The maniac is feared, but also rightly pitied. The professional asylum keepers asserted that they possessed the means by which the maniacal mad might be confined and returned to their reasoned humanity, cured through techniques of appropriate treatment. Here, however, is the layered status: within the confines of the asylum, the maniac must remain frenzied long enough to be rescued and serve the rhetoric of cure, but not so long as to become incurable.

CLASSIFICATION

Once confined, the mad must be appropriately classified if the asylum is to be well regulated and cure assured, so the success of asylums in the United States depended, in large part, upon the rhetoric of classification. Statistical tables included the classifications of insanity recognized by the asylum superintendents and tracked the number of patients admitted by class and by the total in each class who had recovered, been released, or eloped, and who remained. Some reports include more classes of insanity than others, but the primary classifications came to be mania, monomania, melancholy, dementia, and idiocy (these classes were eventually discarded). This classification system also structured the space within the asylum, as inmates of a certain class were removed to the outskirts of the building and those of other classes were housed in a collective center. The classification system that ordered the classes of madness thus shaped both the asylum's architectural structure and its social structure.

This dual class system is perhaps best exemplified in the *Sixteenth Annual Report of the President and Directors of the Western Lunatic Asylum* for 1842. Here the superintendent of the Virginia asylum reiterates what others have articulated: "A classification of the patients, based chiefly on a congeniality of habits, tastes and dispositions, with a due regard to the degree of character of their mental disorder, has been persevered with increasing confidence as to its utility in promoting the contentment and happiness of all concerned." He notes that this kind of classification adds to the order and comfort of the establishment, but has also been used in treatment: "Nothing mortifies a patient more than to be removed for misconduct from a higher to a lower class—whilst on the other hand those are greatly delighted who, in consequence of their merits, are favored in this respect with promotion." Those whose madness was violent or obscene, maniacal in its manifestation, were removed from the community. Those whose madness was quiet and even thoughtful or brooding, of a melancholic nature, were favored with moral treatments that included dinners, amusements, and music.[31]

The moral treatment of violent patients was often used to argue for the importance of accommodating manic classes of patients and to justify additions or new buildings and larger grounds for an asylum. In an *Annual Report of the Managers of the New York State Lunatic Asylum* from 1844, the argument for funding referred to other asylum practices, claiming that "all well organized hospitals for the insane have separate accommodations for the noisy and violent class, and so far removed as not to disturb those who are quiet." The asylum's financial report suggested improvements in accommodating, for instance, the noisy and violent class of patients, who "are now placed in the basement of the present building" but for whom it would be "desirable that other accommodations" be provided.[32] The *Sixteenth Annual Report of the President and Directors of the Western Lunatic Asylum* for 1842 makes the case for additional buildings to house the lower class of patients and thus improve conditions for the better class. The new budget for the year includes intended funding for two buildings, which are smaller and located in the wards north and south of the present buildings, "intended for that class of patients who are noisy, most troublesome, and require close confinement." The present buildings provide for the comfort of the inmates "in a style of neatness, and even elegance, as it regards the better class of patients, which might well compare with that of the best conducted boarding houses in our cities."[33] The practice of confining the maniacs in separate buildings so that the asylum might accommodate fewer violent cases unamenable to moral treatments provided an argument for securing the extraordinary capital required for asylum practices and expansions.

The classification of patients in terms of treatment and accommodations, however, was based as much on class in terms of social status as on symptoms of a particular disorder. All the state asylums declared, in terms similar to that of the *Reports of the Board of Visitors, of the Trustees, and of the Superintendent of the*

New Hampshire Asylum for the Insane for 1843: "It is the object of this institution to extend benefits and advantages to every class of this state."[34]

The report for the Lunatic Asylum of South Carolina in 1842 addresses the issue of social class more directly: "Can the society of the lowest women, whose lives have been lives of infamy, strengthen the virtuous impulses of the youthful girl, who has been educated with the greatest care?"[35] Certainly, the concern for the virtue of a gentleman or a lady who must share accommodations with members of the lower classes and of the worst class of the insane was expressed explicitly to persuade philanthropists and politicians of the necessity of adequate housing and thus for building additional wings. The concern of southern asylums, particularly in Virginia, was aimed, as well, at the lack of separate wards for insane slaves. The Board of Managers of the Eastern Lunatic Asylum in Williamsburg in 1856 argued that Virginia had a responsibility to "this class of persons"—the maniacal slave.[36] In very complex ways, discussions about sex and race in insane asylums were contextualized by national debates about women's rights and the abolition of slavery. The incarceration of the mad in systems of asylum and the violence of the slave system both commented on the prisonlike confinement that revoked civil liberties in a supposed modern democracy. The difference is in classification. With proper care, those of a certain class might be "restored" to their proper classes—whether whore, lady, gentleman, or slave—in a just and utopian society.

In order to improve the class of insanity for those patients who could be restored, the classification of noisy and violent maniacs separately from the rest of the patients was of primary concern. The 1851 report of Williamsburg's Eastern Lunatic Asylum voices the suspicion, though offers no evidence for it, that maniacs who "bay at the moon" like dogs are more likely to be noisy during moonlit nights.[37] Nevertheless, the reports consistently call for separate quarters for patients who require seclusion because of maniacal excitements. The report from New Jersey's State Lunatic Asylum distributed in 1840 "thought proper to make a distinction between the raving Maniac, who may be confined by chains, or other severe restraints, to prevent injury to himself or others, from those of more peaceful disposition."[38]

Although the asylum superintendents' language does very little to delineate the worst class of madness from the lower classes in society, the manic insane are considered harmful to the less severe classes of the insane—not only because of violence or noise, but because of a communicable habit of mind. The managers of the New Jersey State Lunatic Asylum in 1854 state explicitly that classification "is needful for the welfare, and even safety, of the inmates."[39] The report of the managers of the New York State Lunatic Asylum from 1856 describes a certain class of patients who are "of infectious or contagious character." For this class, it would prove beneficial, especially "in cases of acute maniacal disease," to keep the patients in bed, as "such diseases render the general condition of the atmosphere unpleasant and unhealthful." Until cells could be built for the "most violent and disturbed patients" the asylum managers had found it difficult to provide for this "furious and violent" class in a way that they would not disturb the other "parts of the house."[40] This sentiment is repeated in the annual report of the officers of the Vermont Asylum for the Insane in 1860: "In the classification of our patients, we have always endeavored to associate those together who shall be a mutual benefit to each other, or at least, shall not be injurious. Regard is always had to their former condition, education, taste and habits of life. The sensibilities of the insane are frequently rendered more acute by their disease, and require the greatest caution that they are not annoyed by those whose habits are disagreeable and unpleasant."[41] The double meaning here crafts the argument for protection from the chronic and most violent class of insane for the curable and higher class of insane.

The classification of madness within the asylum was an inadequate system. Madness in mania continued to be characterized as both general madness and the worst case of particular madness. Maniacs were separated from the community, allowed to mingle with other classes only after they'd been "restored" from their ravings and could provide suitable dinner company for other inmates. However, mania was never fully reunited with the collective center. The maniac did not possess an appropriately dignified habit of mind, and was thus never fully qualified and always unworthy to participate in the collective madness of the asylum.

Classification of the insane supported a rhetoric that argued for creating and expanding asylums, established practices that distinguished the worst from other kinds of insanity, and crafted mania into a worse class of insanity and a lower class in the social hierarchy, even a potentially infectious condition to be separated and quarantined. In the annual report of the Pennsylvania Hospital for the Insane for 1860, Kirkbride describes this important aspect of asylum design, because classification cannot, in his words, be "over-estimated." Every facility should be designed so that all classes are provided for, "because it is possible for but half a dozen patients to be so totally dissimilar in their natural characteristics, their social positions, and especially in the manifestations of their disease, that no two of them should be together."[42] A report from the Illinois State Hospital for the Insane in 1864 classifies mania as the primary form of insanity and suggests that because of its characteristics—chaotic violence—the asylum is the only resort. Nevertheless, the extremely violent language and action of those afflicted makes their associations with other patients intolerable, and the only beneficial influences are those arising from asylum architecture (as there is no success in regimen, exercise, recreation, or degree of liberty).[43] An 1880 report on the supervision of the asylums in the state of New York emphasizes the importance of separating the "clamorous and dangerous maniacs" who must be "shut up in brick or stone castles" from those insane persons who do not require confinement, and who might be "placed in houses, where they can enjoy a kind of family life."[44]

CURABLE AND CHRONIC CASES

The asylum came into existence, perhaps by more than any other circumstance, out of the claim that insanity could be cured. A new conviction emerged as asylums were erected: correct treatment would provide successful cure. The directors of the Ohio Lunatic Asylum as early as 1839 assured readers of their report: "Already have a number of the most furious maniacs, who were wholly uncontrollable by their friends and a terror to all around them, been fully restored to reason and sent home, while others of a like character are in the progress of cure and will soon be dismissed."[45] Notably, treatment would cure even those who some deemed "incurable"—even the most intractable cases. The "maniac" was thus enrolled to demonstrate the truth of asylum principles and the correctness of their practices. The superintendent for the Virginia Western Lunatic Hospital highlighted medical treatments that worked as cures for mania, describing in an 1836 report a woman admitted to the hospital with "violent paroxysms of derangement, amounting in degree to mania furosia." She appeared rational in no longer than a few weeks. The medical treatment she received in the hospital had prevented any further attacks during her stay. Although it was possible that she might once again suffer from such attacks, the superintendent was certain that "her restoration to her children and friends would prove a powerful barrier to such misfortune."[46]

It was the course of treatment, however, that determined whether cure might be possible. When a patient was considered incurable, the reason might be ill-conceived treatment. When too much time passed before a maniac was confined to an asylum, he or she degenerated. The process is described by the 1840 report of the State Asylum for New Jersey Lunatics: "The furious Maniac, under the pressure of disease, gradually loses one mental faculty after another, until all are lost, and nothing remains of the noble structure, but the mere animal machine. . . . The point at which mania ceases, and idiocy begins, cannot be adequately defined."[47] Reports emphasized that early confinement to an asylum was absolutely necessary, as does, for example, the 1843 report of the New Hampshire Asylum: "The statistics of all the institutions go to show that in the early stage, insanity is as curable as any other disease of equal severity." However, the report also warns that "the hope of recovery fades with its duration until two or three years have elapsed" and the chances of cure are then "very few."[48] Mania was considered curable if treated early but considered the most incurable class of insanity if left untreated for too long. As such, it could be a class of insanity orchestrated to demonstrate the great success of asylum treatment for cure and the continued need for asylum care even once the chance for cure seems to have passed.

Asylum reports acknowledged that readmissions for mania were common— the disease could reoccur years after its first manifestation. The 1843 *Statistical Report of One Hundred and Ninety Cases of Insanity, Admitted into the Retreat near Leeds* by Samuel Hare notes that in this northern England asylum, "all the cases which were admitted more than once were instances of mania."⁴⁹ The maniac was notably among the class of the insane most likely to remain mad. Thus the maniac remains a troubled figure in asylum rhetoric. While the maniac worked as a figure of madness in need of cure and then in need of new architecture and new treatment, the figure also justified chronic care. As noted in the 1851 report of the Eastern Lunatic Asylum in Williamsburg, there must always be some patients "whose whole physical system seems such a chaos of false ideas and transitory though vehement emotions, that the faculty of attention appears lost through the every-varying state of the mind, or through the mighty force of maniacal excitement superadded."⁵⁰ These chronic manic cases came to be viewed as the most incurable. They could merely be "managed." The superintendent for the Illinois State Hospital in 1864 counted the great majority of cases of insanity under the class of acute or chronic mania and noted that these constituted the larger proportion of admissions and had the least chance of recovery.⁵¹

Toward the end of the nineteenth century, asylum reports consistently began to point to custodial care as a further argument that asylum care was essential. The 1876 *Annual Report of the State Board of Charities of the State of New York* could assure readers: "The end of an insane asylum is to aid in curing acute cases, and to make safe and comfortable those in whom the disease has become chronic."⁵² The two types of treatment promised by the end of the nineteenth century, whether for nervous conditions or for organic insanity, are described in the 1896 *Annual Report of the Department for the Insane of the Pennsylvania Hospital*: "The hospital for the insane performs a double function. It receives the first class for medical treatment and the second class for custodial care, together with such medical treatment as will ameliorate and mitigate the disordered condition, whether it be the debility of disease or the paroxysms of maniacal violence."⁵³

Some reports explained the deaths that occurred in asylums by describing the severity of the mania and hinting at the impossibility of cure for these cases. A report of the managers of the New York State Lunatic Asylum in 1873 presented incurable cases in which the patient "failed" or died from pathological insanity inside the asylum, for example, that of "Case 10, Man, age 52": "A week before coming to the asylum, while in church, he became excited, took off his coat, gesticulated violently, talked loudly, and walked rapidly up and down the aisle. The next day he was maniacal and violent, . . . was sleepless, incoherent and boisterous, and rapidly failed." And that of "Case 11: Woman, age 48," became irritable and talkative, followed by maniacal violence, a condition which continued until she finally failed. Cases 12 and 14 detailed very similar scenarios in which the patient became "maniacal" and was described as boisterous, incoherent, noisy, talkative, obscene, and abusive. Both failed after admission. Case 16 described a patient who, "on admission, was wild and maniacal, talked incoherently, was

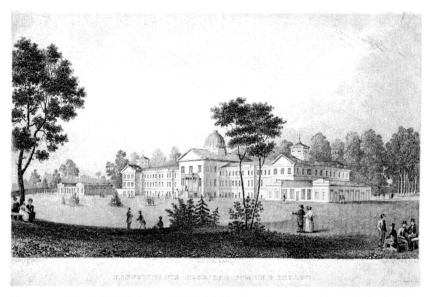

Figure 2.2. Hospital for the Insane, Philadelphia, 1841. *Reproduced by permission from Wellcome Library, London.*

obscene and abusive in speech, was hoarse from constant hallooing," and who died twenty-four days later.[54]

In the memorial for Kirkbride contained in the *Report of the Pennsylvania Hospital for the Insane for the Year 1883*, the superintendent is remembered for the forty-two reports published throughout his service to the hospital. The collection of reports is said to have pointed out the "foundation principles upon which the care and treatment of the insane at this institution were laid forty-three years ago."[55]

As superintendent of the Pennsylvania Hospital for the Insane from 1844 to 1888, Kirkbride emphasized what he took to be the duty of all asylum superintendents: to correct the public sentiment on the matter of asylum treatment for insane persons. He says in his annual report from 1860: "All rightly conducted institutions for the insane become important centers for dispelling prejudices and diffusing sound views in reference to the disease and its treatment—and there can hardly be any part of their mission that is more useful."[56] Kirkbride used his own annual reports to circulate what he thought ought to be the "correct public sentiment." In nearly every one, he states the now universally accepted truth that insanity is an illness, a disease of the organ of the mind. This illness could affect anyone, Kirkbride held, regardless of status or position. Thankfully, insanity, like other illnesses seated in other organs, could be cured. But the promise of cure could be kept only if persons suffering insanity could be quickly confined in hospitals designed specifically for treatment of the insane. Timely confinement of the patient, with appropriate classification of the illness, was necessary if an acute attack were to be cured and chronic illness prevented. Kirkbride's successor at the Pennsylvania Hospital for the Insane credits him, in a memorial, for articulating a philosophy: "Among the indirect results of the publication of these annual reports of the Hospital may be named the diffusion of knowledge of insanity, its causes, treatment and methods of management."[57]

From the inception of the asylum era, mania was the subject of dual logic in arguments about asylum reform. The maniac restored to reason could be enlisted as proof of the success of asylum reform, and thus of the restoration of reason in a reformed republic. But the maniac did not retain his reason; rather he often proved to be incurable and thus served as evidence for the unrealized ideals of all reform. The same frenzied maniac who promised that reformist goals could be realized in asylums also attested to their failure. Throughout the era of asylum, a furious maniac was embattled in the chaotic complexity of "reform"—never himself reformed—rhetorically and materially elusive, unruly, and raging.

ASYLUM MORALS AND METAPHORS

Taken together, the asylum reports detail the principles and practices of asylum superintendents as motivators for commitments from state legislatures, asylum patrons, and public reformers. However, asylum rhetoric did not belong solely to asylum doctors. Articulate conceptions of asylum reform printed in the public press were motivated both by a perceived need for and the accepted progress of asylum treatment, and by new popular attitudes about insanity and trends toward the rejection of asylum methods. While liberal reformists may have provided the public with visions of utopian communities established within asylum walls, support from the public and larger culture cannot be assumed. Certainly, during the asylum's rapid expansion, the profound changes in treatment of insanity would have resulted in changes, as well, in popular attitudes. Unfortunately, asylum reformers inevitably faced the problems as well as the promises of their reforms.

Reform in the insane asylum came to be identified with the new "democratic disease," cast as a new epidemic of madness argued for by statistics indicating the rise of insane cases in U.S. society. Reform movements from abolition to women's rights and proper housing for the poor provided a reminder that the principles of democratic freedom would be challenged by new and disturbing problems. A gap was exposed between what the nation was supposed to be, that is, a city on a hill, and what it was, that is, a republic in need of reform. Lay reformers like Dorothea Dix and literary figures like Edgar Allen Poe produced different kinds of reform rhetoric. Dix remained dedicated to a model of asylum reform based on benevolent and philanthropic premises. Poe rendered "reform" as metaphorical dogma, a dark undercurrent undermining these humanist premises. Asylum reform, as both model and metaphor, stood in for the dizzying heterogeneity of conflicts at play in antebellum America. In strategic ways, then, the figure of the maniac was enacted as the popularized icon of antebellum reform. But he performed as a hybrid figure, defying as well as inciting reform efforts.

Dorothea Dix emerged in the mid–nineteenth century as one of the most prominent participants in the liberal politics of asylum reform. She spent years touring asylums across the country and slowly began to emerge as both a political representative and a public humanitarian on behalf of the insane. In 1843 Dix presented her first endorsement of reform, "Memorial to the Legislature of Massachusetts," in which the maniac plays an integral role in descriptions of almshouses and jails, where conditions for the insane were revealed to be truly appalling. Dix's visit to the Danvers State Insane Asylum in Danvers, Massachusetts, supplies the grist for a typical account from her memorial. Before she even reaches the locale, she hears "wild shouts, snatches of rude songs, imprecations and obscene language" from "the place which was called 'the home' of the forlorn maniac." The young woman from whom these sounds came had once lived as "a respectable person, industrious and worthy." After disappointments and trials shook her mind, "she became a maniac for life." Dix exclaims: "Alas, what a change was here exhibited!" And she describes the woman in more detail: "There she stood, clinging to or beating upon the bars of her caged apartment, the contracted size of which afforded space only for increasing accumulations of filth, a foul spectacle." In Dix's argument for asylum reform the maniac plays an assigned role, true to a predictable performance:

> There she stood with naked arms and disheveled hair, the unwashed frame invested with fragments of unclean garments, the air so extremely offensive, though ventilation was afforded on all sides save one, that it was not possible to remain beyond a few moments without retreating for recovery to the outward air. Irritation of body, produced by utter filth and exposure, incited her to the horrid process of tearing off her skin by inches. Her face, neck, and person were thus disfigured to hideousness. She held up a fragment just rent off. To my exclamation of horror, the mistress replied: "Oh, we can't help it. Half the skin is off sometimes. We can do nothing with her; and it makes no difference what she eats, for she consumes her own filth as readily as the food which is brought her."[58]

Dix publicized her cause in emotional vignettes in proposed legislation. She included these, too, in public appeals to which readers would certainly respond. Dix enlisted the print media, excerpting from the memorial in newspapers and pamphlets, encouraging support from a sympathetic general public. Dix (despite restrictions on her rights to speak due to her gendered status) agitated for support of insane asylums and the deliverance of the maniac from unreasonable suffering. Her very public pleas for benevolent treatment of the frenzied and violent insane won her a national reputation and proved instrumental in the establishment and expansion of asylums across the United States. Dix enrolled the unruly and untamed maniac—one particular entity, which would play a specific and significant role within a wider network of associations—in her emotional argument for state and privately funded asylums, the only humane relief for the horrific suffering of a newly identified U.S. citizenry.

Charles Dickens, traveling the United States, toured the same insane asylums in the same years as Dix. Dickens's *American Notes* offers observations of a New York lunatic asylum that reads as might be expected, given Dix's descriptions. He supplies striking details about the conditions of the asylum and its inmates, depicting the "gibbering maniac" and the ugly horror of his vacant eye, hideous laugh, wild face, and chewed skin and nails. However, when he visits the Insane Asylum at South Boston, he emerges with notably different conclusions. This hospital was "admirably conducted on those enlightened principles of conciliation and kindness, which twenty years ago would have been worse than heretical."[59] Rather than relying upon mechanical restraints, the asylum superintendent gained the trust of his inmates through moral means. Dickens describes daily labor, evening meals, and weekly balls. He credits moral treatment with keeping the violent patients "from cutting the throats of the rest" and describes the immense politeness and dignity of a madwoman who believes herself to be "the lady of the house." He compliments this insane asylum in Boston by finding there a "desire to show some confidence, and repose some trust, even in mad people." In fact, when he visits the Insane Asylum at Hartford, Dickens writes: "I very much questioned within myself, as I walked through the Insane Asylum, whether I should have known the attendants from the patients, but for the few words which passed between the former, and the Doctor, in reference to the persons under their charge."[60] By the time Dickens likened the attendants to the patients, a great many other writers had raised the question as to whether, in fact, the lunatics were running the asylums. Dickens describes a maniac in order to comment on the new democratic system of government in practice; while he seems earnestly impressed with the government of the insane asylum, seeming to suggest that this reformation truly reflected radical U.S. ideas of democracy, he nevertheless stages the maniac to invite apprehension. Dickens repeatedly claims to witness a gulf between democratic reform ideals and their realization in U.S. institutions.

Dickens's various accounts of his visits to these institutions are thought to have been the source of the satire in Edgar Allen Poe's humorous fictional story "The System of Dr. Tarr and Professor Fether," first published in *Graham's Magazine* in November 1845. Poe's narrator (who happens to share certain characteristics with Dickens) is a visitor to an asylum in France, where the so-called moral treatment had been invented. However, in this case, rather than admiring the administration of the asylum, Poe's narrator slowly realizes that he has in fact been duped: the superintendent of the institution has himself become mad, and the lunatics themselves are attending to the place. All the asylum keepers were "first well tarred, then carefully feathered, and then shut up in underground cells." In Poe's story, dinner is interrupted by a screeching fiddle, a bellowing trombone, and dancing that results in pandemonium. Throughout the tale, Poe's estimation of asylum reform is clearly portrayed with a more cynical vision, as he purposefully (even if only temporarily) reverses the positions of doctor and patient, reason and unreason, order and disorder.[61] Certainly, Poe's satire (whether or not it targeted Dickens directly) was aimed explicitly at the ambiguous relationship between reform and reason. In Poe's imagination, monstrosity doubles as normality. But while Poe may be one of the most significant U.S. authors of the nineteenth century to represent obsession with madness in both autobiographical realism and fictionalized sensationalism, he was certainly not the only recognized author to play with the motif of the asylum or madhouse. The nineteenth-century madhouse or asylum, home to reformers and maniacs alike, had become symbolic of the unruly architecture and the disordered reason of social reform.

A.J.H. Duganne, a popular dime novelist, plainly mimicked both Poe's prose and poetry and often shared his politics. Duganne's writing, however, was even darker and his portrayal of the asylum almost absurdly bleak. He describes ghastly asylums in what David Reynolds calls a literature of "dark reform."[62] In the *Knights of the Seal; or, the Mysteries of Three Cities: A Romance of Men's Hearts and Habits*, the reader is cajoled to join the author on a literary tour of the "mad house" in Philadelphia, which "grows wild with horrible cries—laughter that curdles the blood,—low plaintive moans of misery—curses and prayers are mingling" from cells that look like "cages for the wild beasts."[63] When a "furious maniac" escapes, the doctor's "glittering and unblenching glance" fixes upon the other's eyeballs. The doctor—"his eye quailing not"—tames the maniac, who trembles and rushes back to his cell with a cry of fear. Here Duganne employs the gaze described by Tuke, not representative of a soothing or sympathetic treatment but as a means of terrifying control. By the end of Duganne's book, it is the monstrous mad doctor who displays the excessive and murderous frenzy of manic violence. His face is described as ghastly, with livid eyes, twitching nostrils, and a wretched expression of rage. While Duganne, speaking of the maniac in his cell, notes that "there is reason in the mad we know not of," he leaves the "maniacal physician" in the asylum "in the ravings of his madness."[64] For Duganne, the maniac is left neither in a reformed order nor in the house of mad horrors. He is, rather, left without rescue in a story without resolution, contributing to the continuity of unreasonable reform and of madness unreformed.

Pinel himself warned: "The blood of maniacs is sometimes so lavishly spilled, with so little discernment, as to render it doubtful whether the patient or his physician has the best claim to the appellation of a madman."[65] The literary trope at work in Dickens's *American Notes*, in which the mad are indistinguishable from the mad doctor, and that in Poe's "Dr. Tarr and Professor Fether" and Duganne's *Knights of the Seal*, in which the mad doctor and the madmen double, was not unique.[66] Literary fascination with the maniac and the madhouse, with lunacy and its reform, is revealed as a moral and a metaphor for "reform" widely conceived in the work of various men and women of letters. Nathaniel Hawthorne's most spectacular tale of insanity is widely noted to be *House of Seven Gables*, in which a domestic home doubles for a kind of madhouse where (according to a narrator) the characters are all afflicted with lunacy.

In this assemblage of texts, from asylum reports to literary journals and popular press, the new psychiatry is comprised of old models and adorned with old metaphors. The mania that is coordinated in the asylum reports to support a reform movement and the mania that emerges from a nineteenth-century communication culture is that of an overlapping materialized and metaphorized body. The asylum is neither reformed nor fully realized as a medical institution, and mania is never solidified as a scientific object—as a mental illness. The maniac elopes from the asylum, both more and less a real and phenomenal monster. While the maniac possesses an undeniable and iconic reality, his body is a momentarily diverse category. Mania has scattered, multiply transfixed by its cultural salience. The criteria for inclusion in or exclusion from the category "mania" have grown both weaker and stronger.

CONCLUSION

The figure to attend to at the scene in which Pinel removes the chains and looks the maniac in the face is not Pinel. It is the maniac. In Foucault's later writing, while he nevertheless restates his argument that the scene at Bicêtre is the famous scene for "what passes" as the founding scene of modern psychiatry, he puts things differently by emphasizing the surplus power of the patient.[67] Here, Foucault argues that when the maniac manages to exit the asylum doors, there is a new clinical apparatus waiting to capture his neurological body (but which captures, rather, the sexual body beneath). Foucault describes the absence of a diagnosable body. Perhaps, however, what provides the maniac with his surplus of power is not only this absence but a network of linkages that have captured his perverse, destructive, excessive, devilish gestures (the sexual body only one of multiple pathological bodies).

After the maniac has eloped from the asylum and its revolutionary reform practices, he is secured by the "print reform" and "communication revolution." When he is returned to the public sphere, a source of endless symbolic and metaphorical practices, he returns as a maniac at once rhetorical and material. New forms of the mania classification, from references in letters and journals to "piano mania" and "the mania for yellow curls," testify to the multiplication of manic events. Of particular concern in the mid–nineteenth century was a mania for moneymaking. The *Journal of Insanity* published an editorial on this topic in 1849, noting that "this disease" has prevailed in almost every age, and "at present, there is no institution for the insane that does not present some instances of

persons having become deranged in mind, from indulging fallacious expectations of great wealth." The author warns that bank excitement and speculating
excitement have "furnished the Asylum with inmates," and cites specific
schemes that have caused speculation excitement and insanity as warnings
against entertaining false hope for great riches.[68]

One cause of insanity in the new democratic society was thus a maniacal or
monomaniacal pursuit of undue excitements and unrealizable hopes for the
"wicked dollar" in a capitalist marketplace. Indeed, asylum reports that classified
madness also discussed its causes. The first was constitutional: a patient may
have a predisposition toward insanity, perhaps because of heredity. The second
was an exciting and external influence more difficult to determine, but among
the external influences were financial losses due to the excessive pursuit of riches.
Asylums were built to reflect a nation restored to its reason, to its revolutionary
ideals. Nevertheless, these institutions aligned its maniacs in networks that did
not restore social order or protect an ordered citizenry.

Asylum practices in the eighteenth century have been described by Benjamin
Reiss as "something of a spectator sport." Arguing that Foucault cannot tell us
the whole story of the asylum as battlefield, Reiss cites what he sees to be a
"dialectical tension between the institutional processing of culture and the cultural processing of the institution."[69] What has been demonstrated in this chapter is that asylum practices enrolled mania in doubled and multiple justifications
for creating and preserving the utopian dream of moral treatment: confinement,
classification, and cure. Reform was always a utopian dream and a dystopian
nightmare. The maniac enacted these dreams and nightmares and was aligned
by them—the icon of the asylum, of both the cure in reformation and the
chronicity of unreason. Too, those same practices of the asylum regime and its
maniacs were enacted differently by critical perceptions of the public outside
the asylum. Always there was risk of commitment. And so the maniac today
remains an iconic figure, appearing in some of our most public spaces—not only
in literature but also in popular culture, in television and film—as a real threat
to society and a symbolic (because we know it only momentarily) return to
stability.

CHAPTER 3

MIDWESTERN MANIA

GENETICS IN THE HEARTLAND

Thus there is clear evidence that there is a genetic factor at work in the affective disorders and most particularly in bipolar affective disorder.

—George Winokur, *Mania and Depression*

In the asylum, madness was transmittable, mania inherited, and chronic mental illness incurable. Mania could be transferred, at least in the sense that the sufferer would badly influence the quieter and calmer class of patients, and so must be confined. The rhetoric of inheritance as cause for mania justified the label "incurable" and the need for custodial care. The shift from a nineteenth-century concept of heredity, to the early twentieth-century concept of genetics, to the late twentieth-century materialization of genomics shaped the rhetoric of etiology, classification, and treatment of mania. For a time in the early to mid–twentieth century, the eugenics movement used heredity to call for the elimination (by way of sterilization) of contaminants to the population, including the inherited traits of madness. Later in the twentieth century, mania was studied extensively as part of family history research, which attempted to provide both a clinical and a genetic etiology that might ensure some diagnostic validity for the illness and thus guide better prevention as well as treatment. At the same time, another mania was coming into being—one that was genetic and biological. By the end of the century, mania had come to be a set of clinical criteria that was visibly performed both as bodily symptoms and as biological material, nearly visible, as a molecule, within a biomedical model of molecular genetics.

This chapter traces the coming into being of mania as defined by old notions of heredity and the emergence of a new model of genomics that had yet to secure authority. I move through "different times within the present"—the outdated, intersecting, transient, and current concepts of heredity, genetics, and genomics—to trace the multiple ways in which mania has been mobilized as both the observed symptoms of madness in a diagnosis and the matter made visible by a DNA molecule.[1]

When George Winokur accepted the position of chair of the Department of Psychiatry at the University of Iowa's College of Medicine in 1971, he visited what was then the University of Iowa Psychopathic Hospital, where he found a basement full of "a gold mine of information."[2] The hospital had kept a record for every admitted patient since it had opened in 1921. Records for thousands of patients were easily accessible, and each record included not only admission charts, progress notes, and discharge summaries, but also typed transcripts of interviews—all of sufficient detail and quality to begin the design of what is now referred to as the Iowa 500 study of familial relationships in depression, bipolar disorder, and schizophrenia. In addition, because so few people in the state of Iowa migrated from home, Winokur imagined he would be able to conduct interviews with discharged patients or with family members to determine family history.

The Iowa 500 study used patient records and family study methodology to investigate whether the presence of an affective disorder in one family member would make it more likely for there to be an affective disorder in other members of the family. This study was important, in particular, because it used both clinical evaluation of symptomology based on recorded observations of patients and study of family background to determine the etiology of the disorder. Winokur believed that symptomology was important to diagnosis, but that the addition of clear family history would indicate whether an individual might be at higher risk. For Winokur, psychiatric genetics was primarily a biological problem. He was convinced, in fact, that a positive genetic factor would "suggest an unequivocal biological factor."[3] The Iowa 500 study has been described in more than one review as a "landmark study" and "pioneering work." Upon Winokur's death in 1996, he was memorialized for this work: his "linkage studies since the 1960s paved the way for the current state of the field of psychiatric genetics."[4]

Heredity as a modern biological concept did not exist until the last third of the nineteenth century. Staffan Müller-Wille and Hans-Jörg Rheinberger have documented an "ontological drift" that transposed "heredity" as a complex metaphor of inheritance of family holdings to "heredity" as a biological concept referring to traits or dispositions.[5] According to Müller-Wille and Rheinberger, the radical drift from analogy to biology occurred primarily within the medical discourse of madness. The status of mania from general madness to something material and molecularized occurred during the critical shift from the era of asylum to this new genetic psychiatry. This new status for mania was aligned with similar shifts in the new psychiatry from the notion of "heredity" to the more complex "genetic rationality."[6] The start of genetic rationality launched new practices of experimentation and record keeping. References to hereditary disease from the mid– to the late nineteenth century were used to account for chronic disorders, like mania, that were deemed unpreventable or incurable.

These were hereditary defects. For the psychological eugenics movement, the study of hereditary defects was a major breakthrough in the application of scientific method to the problems of mental illness that eugenicists believed were contributing to a degenerating human race. People suffering mental illness who were gathered in large populations in mental institutions made good subjects for eugenic study. Further, in such state institutions researchers could trace heritable patterns and keep track of large amounts of data amassed in the records of such large populations.

Rather than begin, as one easily could, at Cold Spring Harbor Laboratory—founded in 1890, the home of the Eugenics Record Office from 1910 to 1944, now a renowned laboratory for research in genomics and bioinformatics—I begin with the state of Iowa, its rigorous participation in the project of eugenics, the Iowa 500 study, and my own participation in the genomic study of mania. While Cold Spring Harbor may have been the official central site for the eugenics movement, the practices of a eugenics ideology played out across the country, certainly in the midwestern states like Iowa. After a strong eugenics program faded, George Winokur's renowned work in psychiatric genetics in the Iowa 500 studied genetic linkages for bipolar disorder. Finally, I offer some details regarding research in molecular genetics in which I participated. The purpose of this project was to identify the "specific genetic variations that influence BD [bipolar disorder] susceptibility."[7] Indeed, the primary researchers suggested that they had replicated previous findings and had likely identified one of these "variations." The conversations in subsequent genomic research necessarily engage with questions regarding mania and its multiplicity, with global genomewide association studies and with consequent personalized medicine.

HEREDITY AND INHERITANCE

The argument that physicians needed to account for their failure to treat chronic disease—in particular, mysterious diseases with late and sudden onset and development, especially those like mania—is left over from asylum medicine and remains familiar. In the 1855 volume of the *Iowa Medical Journal*, D. L. M'Gugin of the Iowa Medical Department advocates for the "common sense view" that for certain diseases, including insanity, "persons are born with the disease and are diseased during life, and this may be extended through from the cradle to the grave, and yet not evince internal changes, but will still transmit the material to their offspring, whose different relations to the external world will exhibit changes such as their grandparents evinced in their lives." Also in that year's *Iowa Medical Journal*, M'Gugin continues the discussion of heredity among the insane within what could come to be known as a eugenics philosophy. Here, he describes the "degeneracy of the race." Regarding this state of affairs, M'Gugin advocates for prohibiting the consummation of marriage for people with latent disposition to insanity. He describes the terrible evil in cases where insanity is handed from parent to child, as nothing can equal the intensity of this affliction. He asserts that when hereditary cases are reported to the superintendents of lunatic asylums, there is a need "by some civil regulation" to prevent the dread disease and to save civilization from further infliction.[8]

Asylum superintendents in the nineteenth century emphasized documentation and kept records and statistics for patients who were restored and for those who suffered from chronic conditions. Not every cause for madness was considered to be heritable, and heredity appeared in asylum reports in the same list as environmental causes. The report of the officers of the Iowa Hospital for Insane for fiscal 1866–1867 included a table of reported causes of insanity with the number of cases for each, for example, "disappointments" triggered 21 cases of insanity. A list of causes points to quite a few possibilities: "business anxieties" (27), "jealousy" (4), "domestic troubles" (58), "religious excitement" (45), "uterine disease" (3), and "novel-reading" (1). Heredity appears as the cause for 22 cases of insanity.[9] The 1874 report of the Hospital for the Insane at Independence, Missouri, also lists causes and total cases for each. Ten years later, similar causes reappear on the list: intemperance, domestic difficulty, disappointed affections, close attention to study, and religious excitement. While the cited causes of insanity remain numerous, by this time heredity is blamed for the highest number of cases.[10]

The superintendents' tabulations of cases of madness transmitted by heredity provided the data to identify patients who suffered from a heritable and thus incurable disease. Mania, in particular, was hereditary. An article in the *Iowa Medical Journal* from 1895 states explicitly that the cause of both mania and melancholy is an inherited disposition and that the greatest influence on prognosis is heredity. For those with the prognosis of predisposition, or heredity, cure is seldom permanent.[11] As madness was coming to be less a vague idea about inheritance of character, mania was coming to be a specific heritable disease that could be documented in statistical tables and recorded as data. In 1914 the causes of insanity and number of supposed cases in all Iowa asylums or hospitals were gathered into a single document; heredity was separated from environmental factors as a single cause and placed in table number 201, "Forms of Insanity and Heredity of Patients." According to the table, there were 528 cases of manic depression, one of the highest populations of the mentally ill. Of these, those in the class "maniacal state" numbered 227. Also included in this table were statistics for the number of cases in which family members—grandparents, parents, brothers or sisters, uncles or aunts, cousins, and children—were also hospitalized for maniacal insanity: 11 grandparents, 37 parents, 37 counted brothers or sisters, 46 uncles or aunts, 13 cousins, and 2 children. Of the 227 patients identified as experiencing maniacal insanity, then, the total number of patient family members hospitalized for the same type of insanity is 146.[12]

Once a case had been made for madness as an inherited trait and mania as a cause for hereditary defect, the eugenic pronouncements concerning the danger of mania to individuals and the consequences of allowing madness to spread through the population became more prevalent. Iowa's *Bulletin of State Institutions* published in January 1922 from the proceedings of the quarterly conference for officers of the institutions included fewer statistics and more discussion regarding the subject of insanity and "adverse heredity."[13] In the bulletin, an article entitled "Inherited Insanities" by R. A. Stewart, the superintendent at Independence State Hospital, addresses the importance of heredity to a "common type" of insanity: manic-depressive insanity. Stewart argues that there are families showing a "preponderance" of this illness. He refers to a study in Zurich which found that "defective heredity is the most important cause occurring in from 70 to 80 per cent of cases" of manic-depressive illness.[14] Stewart cites other physicians, all of whom agree that the "essential feature" in the cause of manic-depressive insanity is a "constitutional predisposition, which is believed to be hereditary" (130). The "defective constitution" of an individual may appear before onset of the manic-depressive insanity: peculiarity, excitability, and moodiness. Regardless, the point is made explicitly that in manic-depressive insanity, "the disease almost always appears independently of external causes" (129). Within segments of the eugenics movement, general madness was thought to be a dangerous hereditary trait, and madness as mania particularly so.

In this bulletin, as the topic of heredity is taken up in several papers, discussion of adverse heredity is introduced in arguments that suggest that reducing the problem of heredity—ridding the human family of defectiveness—is the largest problem the Iowa institutions' officers now face. In several papers, matters of "adverse heredity" provide the basis for discussion of psychological eugenics—and the "campaign against degeneracy" (155). Psychological eugenics was practiced nationwide, but it was a particularly robust movement in Iowa, where it launched popular campaigns: Iowa was the ninth state to pass a sterilization law. It was also one of the few to actually carry out sterilization laws. Iowa's first eugenics law, passed on July 4, 1911, appears on the Acts of the Thirty-fourth General Assembly of Iowa (1911) as Chapter 129. The law reads:

An Act to prevent the procreation of habitual criminals, idiots, feeble-minded, and imbeciles. Be it enacted by the General Assembly of the State of Iowa: Section 1. Unsexing of Criminals, Idiots, Lunatics, etc. That it shall be the duty of the managing officer of each public institution in the state . . . to annually, or oftener, examine into the mental or physical condition of the inmates of such institutions, with a view to determining whether it is improper to allow any of such inmates to procreate. The surgical superintendent of such institution shall judge whether procreation by any such inmate would produce children with a tendency to disease, crime, insanity, feeble-mindedness, idiocy, or imbecility. If there is no probability that the condition of any such inmate so examined will improve to such an extent as to render procreation by any such inmate advisable ... then the surgeon of the institution shall perform the operation of vasectomy or ligation of the Fallopian tubes, as the case may be, upon such person.[15]

To apply Iowa's first eugenics law of 1911, the managing officers of state hospitals and institutions were to document those cases of mental illness (along with feeblemindedness and alcoholism) that were caused by heredity—and to determine by examination whether or not mental conditions made it likely that offspring would be likely victims of insanity. Cases in which mental degeneracy was considered to be caused by hereditary taint presented a danger to the entire population, and thus sterilization was the obvious and appropriate solution. By 1929 a eugenics committee, including the medical director of the Iowa Psychopathic Hospital and the superintendents of all four state hospitals for the insane, were appointed for the purpose of creating legislation to reduce the inheritable "stock defect" shown particularly in insanity.[16]

Henry Laughlin, who was born in Iowa in 1880 and later attended Iowa State College, is considered to be the principal force behind the passage of sterilization laws around the country. Laughlin was easily recruited by Charles Davenport, crusader for eugenic research and policy in the United States and founder of a eugenics research station at Cold Spring Harbor in New York. Laughlin served at Cold Spring Harbor as superintendent and then the director in charge of the Eugenics Record Office, a branch of the Department of Genetics for the Carnegie Institute of Washington, D. C., from its origin in 1910 until 1940. He was a prolific writer who carried out far-reaching educational programs, establishing him as an expert and as a popularizer for eugenics. Laughlin used visual display as well as print to popularize his ideas for reducing defects in the race. The first live "better breeding" exhibit to emphasize the importance of good marriage was staged at the 1911 Iowa State Fair. A display highlighting a "Better Baby Contest" advised parents to consider hereditary traits before they "scored" a baby. Organized eugenics exhibits became common sights at state fairs around the country. The Better Baby Contest became a traveling Fitter Family contest. In this context, mental illness, and manic depression in particular, came to be a different kind of threat to society. Laughlin, concerned with family pedigree for those classified with the manic-depressive defect, offers a pedigree chart that demonstrates the heredity of manic depression. (Figure 3.1)

According to Laughlin: "There is no class of anti-social individuals more definitely and sharply marked off from the general social body, so far as their principles of conduct are concerned, than the insane class," which specifically included manic depression.[17] Figure 3.1 shows a eugenics "flashcard" depicting two individuals labeled as "Mania Depressus." Those classified with madness not only posed a potentially violent threat to themselves and others, but now their mania was a specific illness that could be transmitted through physical means to future generations, contaminating entire populations. Mania again becomes

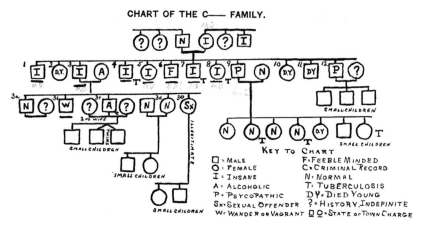

Figure 3.1. Pedigree chart of the C___ family, Cold Spring Harbor Laboratory, 1911. *Courtesy of American Philosophical Society.*

unstable. The risks of heredity were too great. If not confronted, if not "bred out" of the human race, those tainted with mania would breed, multiply, and contribute to the "degeneracy" of the entire species.

GENETIC RATIONALITY

Psychological eugenics survived the first four decades of the twentieth century but was altered significantly in the course of the Nazi eugenics program, and after World War II quickly came to be regarded (at best) as a discredited approach to heredity. Nevertheless, during the mid–twentieth century, the function of heritability in common psychiatric diseases continued to be a site of scientific inquiry. After DNA as a potential carrier of genetic material gained ontological authority, but prior to the period of transformation from genetics to genomics, sustained techniques for family studies coordinated new efforts to attribute trait variance in psychiatric diseases to inheritance. Family heritability studies during the second half of the twentieth century emerged in what Phillip Thurtle calls a culture of "genetic rationality."[18] Important in this genetic rationality culture were new practices in record keeping and data processing that could track heritable patterns, including mania, from one generation to another across large populations. The collection and categorization of data included not only a system for accounting for individuals and family histories, but also the manifestation of information processing: new kinds of record keeping, new possibilities for data analysis, new ways for generating institutional memory, and emerging circuits of communication.

George Winokur and his collaborator, Ming T. Tsuang, drew on this new genetic rationality when they used psychiatric records at the University of Iowa

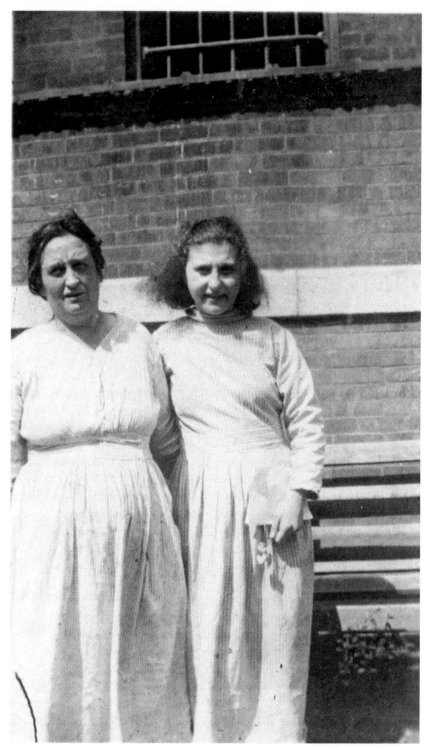

Figure 3.2. "Mania depressus," Cold Spring Harbor Laboratory, circa 1922.
Courtesy of American Philosophical Society.

Psychopathic Hospital to begin their Iowa 500 study in 1971. Their procedures for collecting data and computerizing information depended on "well-designed data management procedures" that would be "used for many years to come."[19] The Iowa 500 study was conceived in 1971, published in pieces in journal articles by 1975, and printed in a full manuscript with an introduction in 1996. The patients chosen for this study had been admitted to the hospital between 1934 and 1940 (with some selected through 1944 to collect the desired number of patients diagnosed with schizophrenia). The total number of cases selected included 100 bipolar patients, 225 unipolar patients, and 200 schizophrenic patients. The selected cases proved to be acceptable because the records were complete, elaborate, and included a personal clinical examination. According to Winokur, the work could be accomplished at the Iowa Hospital because "Iowa has a relatively stable population, and we didn't believe that patients would migrate outside the state to any great extent," so discharged patients and their relatives could be located and follow-up interviews scheduled. Winokur himself argued that this study was "one of the first large-scale psychiatric surveys performed in the United States" (42, 19).

Before Winokur could proceed with his family background study, however, he needed to identify those cases from the thousands stored for which he could confirm an earlier diagnosis of mania or depression. In the description of the study, Winokur emphasizes that he would be able to develop a clinical picture of mania by "capturing" the real symptoms as exhibited by real people. It was therefore important to include in each case the transcripts from patient interviews recorded during their time at the hospital, which detailed the patient-physician dialogue and documented the patient's behavior during the interview. These interviews, with personal examinations and doctors' notes, provided the information Winokur needed to confirm or dismiss an initial diagnosis of mania. After combining the information from all the cases, Winokur was able to identify a shared cluster of symptoms and begin to build valid clinical criteria for mania. However, the interviews reproduced in the study, as Winokur presents them, appear very much like a collage of madness. The figure of the maniac exposed in selected excerpts here will spill over into the clinical picture of mania.

In an interview transcribed in April 1935, a woman identified as JMM, diagnosed with mania, asserted repeatedly that she was not sick, was not in need of rest, and had nothing wrong with her mind. JMM was admitted, according to the history, due to her pressured talk, mood lability, and periods of manic excitement. She was identified as a single white woman who was "over-active, talkative, belligerent, uncooperative, sarcastic" (41). According to the case file, follow-up interviews with JMM became increasingly difficult; her mood was described as elevated, and excited, as well as "silly." During interviews, she threw her shoes and held her head under a water faucet as if she might drown herself.

The admission interview of a second patient diagnosed with mania, AFM, was recorded in December 1937. AFM experienced "a mental illness of periodic type" (74), marked by periods of extreme excitement with bizarre ideas about mental telepathy. AFM describes one of her telepathic experiences: "I feel that through telepathy he was able to contact my thoughts in that direction" so that "just as two wires cross so might our thoughts cross. It wasn't a work language but a thought language." AFM claims her telepathic experiences have been shared, citing for example, a gentleman who nodded to her "verifying that he had my thought" (77).

A series of interviews took place with a boy referred to as RUM, again with the diagnosis of mania. In records dated October 1936, the boy's speech was consistently noted as pressured, loud, argumentative, rambling, and rhyming: "That reminds me of a picture with Joe. E. Brown. He pulled a house with an earthwork tractor; the people in it thought an earthquake had occurred; that reminded me of Quaker Oats, quake, afraid. That is why I was startled. I called Father Goretzsky 'Foxey' because his initials are FX" (84–85). RUM expressed a desire to travel to Washington to plead with the president to stop the war in Spain, and wished even to go to Spain himself to stop the war. When asked about going to Spain, he talked about fighting rebels in a gang. In his room, RUM defecated in his bed, and he talked openly of this act.

The interviews depict manic patients as excited and talkative, with rhyming speech. They are silly and overactive. Delusions are persistent. These patients are also loud, obnoxious, and sarcastic. At the extremes, they are uncooperative and belligerent, potentially violent. And like the mad in the asylum, RUM has become nearly the obscene and animalistic maniac in the unapologetic and inappropriate defecation in his room. Winokur eventually reassembled these acts of madness into clinical criteria. As he collected interviews and cases, he experimented with criterion-based psychiatric diagnosis, providing a prototype for what would later become institutionalized as the DSM-III. In his 1991 publication *Mania and Depression: A Classification of Syndrome and Disease*, Winokur notes the importance of observing symptoms to develop clinical criteria for diagnosis, but also notes the lack of sufficient means for actually "showing" an illness.

In *Mania and Depression*, Winokur states that he will adopt the "medical model" for developing diagnostic validity in classifying mania and the other affective disorders. A clinical description *and* the family history would be important. The clinical description would include behavior, a cluster of symptoms. His clinical description of the manic syndrome accounts for every possible way the illness might be enacted but continues to evoke madness. He notes that "patients with mania show heightened sexuality and are generally uninhibited" and describes symptoms such as rapid thinking, racing thoughts, and pressured speech, along with both euphoria and irritable mood. In addition, mania might be enacted with increased alcohol intake, insomnia, distractibility, and delusions or hallucinations (among a much longer list).[20] This familiar cluster of words is enough to sustain the connection between madness and mania, even in the clinical description. And yet "mania" also comes to be connected to the language of a medical model of biological disease applied to psychiatry. Winokur wrote for much of his career on the importance of correct classification of the affective disorders, suggesting that there are both proximal etiologies, which are pathophysiologies and symptomatic, and distal etiologies, which are genetic and familial.

Although mania has always been described as a cluster of symptoms, Winokur's research argued that a clinical picture of mania that also includes a family history might demonstrate a known genetic factor. Mania had become "more than one" in the sense that it had yet to exclude a mad reality, although it had accumulated a clinical reality and (almost) a genetic reality. Winokur argued for the potential for discovering diagnostic criteria for psychiatric illnesses that have been validated by family background studies. This held value for both diagnosis and potential prevention: "Coming from a family with one of these illnesses puts a person at risk for the same illness; therefore we could predict the onset of such an illness with increased certainty." And "if we had a good idea of how to prevent such psychiatric illnesses, . . . we could bring into play preventive measures to ward off the illness." Then, Winokur suggests, "it may be possible in a stepwise fashion to approach a specific gene involved in transmission and describe the *modus operandi* of that particular gene."[21] The reason to follow up with family history is to trace mania and its potential "genetic factor"—a specific gene.

Winokur remained convinced from the time he started his work on the Iowa 500 study in 1971 to his last attributed work published in 1998 that family history and family study methods were promising avenues for finding the genetic basis of affective disorders.[22] He continued to work with research teams to determine whether mutations in DNA might be involved in the transmission of bipolar disorder, mania moved from one site to another—from the clinical picture to the molecular gene. A publication Winokur coauthored, published in 1997, traced the attempt to determine whether a mitochondrial DNA abnormality—specifically a deletion in mtDNA—was implicated in affective disorders and in bipolar disorder in particular. The results did not support the hypotheses. It appeared that the potential for contribution to heredity and transmission of bipolar disorder in mitochondrial DNA was highly complex and considerably unpredictable.

As mania travels between these sites, from the cluster of symptoms to the genetic material responsible for its transmission, questions arise. What now counts as mania? Is it located in its clinical picture? Can it be recognized in DNA? Indeed, it may be in both. Madness and mania hang together in these medical sites—for now. The "biomedical model" of psychiatry has come to frame theories about the etiology and hence the treatment of mental illness. If this model can account adequately for a brain that is manic and provide predictive and preventative practices, mania may pass away. If it is enacted neither as a clinical picture nor as a genetic mutation, it may appear in some as yet to be imagined alternative configuration, for better, worse, or both. Of course, if the clinical picture remains while the genetic mutation passes away, mania might also remain stubbornly mad.

Genes and Genomics

The term "gene" was first adopted in 1909, but its introduction came with the claim that whether the gene was hypothetical or material was of little consequence. Classical genetics in the early twentieth century, predating the most recent success in molecular genetics and genomics, treated genes as real, but as abstract and invisible "action" underlying aspects of heritability. After DNA was discovered and the gene emerged as a molecular concept, it came to be a stronger unit. New methods of molecular genetics and advanced technologies of "observation" transformed the invisible gene to the visible molecule. Genes may or may not have existed, but the DNA molecule is really there. The discourse regarding genetics commonly used the idea of genetic action to promise the discovery of a "gene for" specific traits. The "gene for" rhetoric handled heredity and inheritance in our genetic makeup as the unifying building blocks that would give us a picture of human life—and uncover the blueprint that would determine our futures. Finding a hereditary "gene for" bipolar disorder could interrupt the coordination between madness and mania, and bring mania into an alternative existence.[23] If such a gene could be found, new practices and technologies might be developed for screening genetic markers and manipulating the cause of the illness. The powerful language of the gene—accompanied by mythical and believable explanations of inheritable traits—comes into being as an ontological basis for what is real. As powerful as the classical genetics (what is now sometimes referred to as "transmission genetics") promise was to link a particulate gene to bipolar disorder, the gene for search lost strength when other genetic approaches framed classical genetics as too simplistic. Using the methods of molecular genetics, genomics research looks not only for individual genes-for, but also for the relationship between multiple genes that might regulate genetic expression as well as protein function. The gene now had the power to turn madness from a collage of symptoms into bipolar disorder, a genetic manipulation of DNA, and then into a relationship among multiple molecules. Along the way, madness as an inherited trait begins to pass away, and mania multiplies in another molecular direction.

Beginning in 1988, the U.S. National Institutes of Mental Health sponsored the Genetics Initiative for Bipolar Disorder Consortium (Bipolar Consortium). In 2006, a group of researchers from the Bipolar Consortium convened to conduct a genomewide association study of bipolar disorder. From 1990 to 2008, the Bipolar Consortium has amassed more than 3,500 subjects with bipolar disorder.[24] The consortium has initiated several important research studies, producing the first findings to determine gene variations associated with bipolar disorder. The University of Iowa has participated in this consortium, along with at least eleven additional extramural sites. The program began with the purpose of building a national database with a large enough sample of interviews and cell lines to identify vulnerability genes for bipolar disorder.

The research group published a paper in *Molecular Psychiatry* in August 2009 titled "Genome-Wide Association of Bipolar Disorder in European American and African American Individuals." This study claimed to have replicated previous research, thus providing additional support for previously reported findings. The study implicated the ANK3 gene and the 15q14 chromosome with increased risk for bipolar disorder. In addition, discussion of the results argued that some SNPs (single-nucleotide polymorphisms) indicated strong enough associations in multiple genetic regions as to warrant more attention. The study introduces its review of current research of genetic research for bipolar disorder (BD) by noting that "the development of genome-wide association (GWA) study designs and analysis methods have made it possible to search for multiple genetic variations underlying a condition like BD" (756). The authors identify several genetic regions of interest and argue: "Our GWA study of BD provides some support for previous findings that variation in ANK3 and at 15q14 influence BD susceptibility" but conclude that "it is likely . . . that the majority of the genetic variations that influence BD remain yet to be discovered" (762).

I volunteered to participate in this study. The final number of subjects used in the study was 1,001 European Americans and 345 African Americans. I was screened and asked for detailed information about myself, my parents, and my siblings. I completed the "Diagnostic Interview for Genetic Studies Self-Report" (DIGS) and gave informed consent for phlebotomy. Whether my information was selected from among the final collection of sample subjects, I do not know.

A representative for the study came to my home to collect data for my DIGS. After a few warm-up questions, the real interview started: "What is the most responsible job you have ever held? Have you been in psychotherapy or in counseling? Have you ever been admitted to a hospital or day hospital because of problems with your mood, emotions, or how you were acting? Have you ever taken medications for your nerves or any emotional or mental problems?" Easy enough questions. Those that followed were slightly more specific, but not particularly surprising. "Did you ever have a period when you were unusually irritable, clearly different from your normal self so that you would shout at people or start fights or arguments? Have there been times when you felt much more energetic than usual and needed less sleep than usual? Did you experience racing thoughts or pressure to keep talking? Were you over-confident? Did you make unrealistic plans?" Of course, I did. Who hasn't?

The diagnostic interview reminded me of my first psychiatric intake. I needed to be identified as a subject with bipolar disorder if my genes were to be included in this study. There were a lot of questions in the interview. Or maybe I was giving a lot of answers. The characteristics—the symptoms—of bipolar disorder were pinned down in this set of ten questions:

- Were you uncharacteristically impulsive? Did you experience increased activity or increased talkativeness? Were you more active than usual either sexually, socially, or at work, or were you physically restless?
- Were you more talkative than usual or did you feel pressure to keep on talking?
- Did your thoughts race or did you talk so fast that it was difficult for people to follow what you were saying?
- Did you feel you were a very important person, or that you had special powers, plans, talents, or abilities?
- Did you have more trouble than usual concentrating because your attention kept jumping from one thing to another?
- Did you do anything that could have gotten you into trouble—like buy things, make business investments, have sexual indiscretions, drive recklessly?
- During this episode was there at least a week when these symptoms that you report above were present most of the time?
- Would you say your behavior was provocative, obnoxious, arrogant, or manipulative enough to cause problems for your family, friends, or co-workers?
- Were you so excited that it was almost impossible to hold a conversation with you?
- During this episode, did you have beliefs or ideas that you later found out were not true? Like believing that you had powers and abilities others did not have? Or that you had a special mission, perhaps from God? Or that someone was trying to harm you? How certain were you?

There were the symptoms of madness classified as mania. The questions were, as to be predicted, "textbook," although not from a single textbook but from them all. By mobilizing layers of textbook symptoms and traces of Greek origins, madness had become meaningful in the "Diagnostic Interview for Genetic Studies" in the new study of genomics. Mania continues to come into the being in more than one way.

The interview questions firmed up the classification of mania by naming its maniacal symptoms: impulsivity, inappropriate sexual activity, pressured speech, racing thoughts, grandiose thinking, lack of focus, recklessness, obnoxious behavior, boisterousness, or arrogance. Delusional, and dangerous. At the time I took the survey, I needed to think about a couple of these questions. Cause problems? I guess so—yes. Indiscreet and reckless? I suppose that would be true. Obnoxious? Likely. Special powers and abilities? Well, ... once. Excited? Absolutely. Suddenly, and again, I was not bipolar, I was manic, a maniac, mad. Rereading the list of questions with the symptoms emphasized, I can't help but conjure Kraepelin's photograph of a maniac.

But the mania I was participating in at this setting was different. I was participating by consent in a research program I hoped would eventually create new kinds of knowledge about bipolar disorder and thus new kinds of ontological possibilities for people with bipolar disorder. I was part of an investigation to turn a mutation into a cause, a diagnosis, and a treatment. I was a part of an effort to make mania the cluster of symptoms into mania as molecule. A different story was being told. This was my mania at the molecular level. And yet, the criteria for inclusion in the study ensured that madness would follow mania into the molecule. Madness makes the interactions between mania and its molecular information possible, at least for now, because potential study participants must be identified as mad—maniacs—to be included in genomic studies of bipolar disorder. The study of the genomic associations with bipolar disorder continue to play with the tension between the symptoms of mania as madness, as defined by a diagnostic test, and the recognition of bipolar disorder at the molecular level at the ANK3 region, in sample DNA transformed into data.

CONCLUSION: MANIA AS (IM)MATERIAL

By submitting to this new enactment of mania, however, I had also become entangled in the labor, the instruments, and the material of genomics—the "politics of life itself."[25] After I was interviewed, I was bled, that is, samples of my blood were taken. I signed the consent form and so, perhaps, if my samples passed quality control, my blood would have been sent to the Broad Institute Center for Genotyping and Analysis. Here DNA quantity is checked, sample quality is assessed, genotyping is carried out, and allele calling is completed. I understand none of these processes. If, in fact, my sample did pass through these various stages, it—or the information it carried—likely still exists, somewhere, in some form. According to the supplementary material included with the article, "all genotypic and phenotypic data for the BiGS subjects, as detailed above, are available through the GAIN dbGAP database (http://www.ncbi.nlm.nih.gov/gap) and the NIMH data repository (http://www.nimhgenetics.org)."[26] These data resources continue to be used by academic researchers globally for the study of bipolar disorder. They are also used by biotechnology and pharmaceutical companies. It is no revelation that there are databases and repositories storing biological materials, and that these materials are circulated around a network of medical and technological nodes. Here mania is multiplied again, now collected and circulated as bioinformation. The "wet" or fluid biological material—the blood and the DNA—is made immaterial, encoded into a database.

My bioinformation may be stored in some repository, awaiting the next circulation. Likely that circulation will move this bioinformation well beyond the Midwest and onto a network of global scale. For some critics, my manic gene, though gifted by consent, has been commodified in the global market, at least to some extent, in a transaction of biological identity. And so I have participated in a postgenomic biocapitalism by interacting with practices of tissue economics.

Researchers at the National Human Genome Research Institute and the National Institutes of Health have described "the current explosion of genomewide association studies" as the most important advances relevant to personalized medicine.[27] These studies are based on the search of gene-disease relationships using large numbers of individuals and searching for statistical associations between the most common form of genetic variation and single nucleotide polymorphisms (SNPs). Association studies have been described as genomic medicine—genomewide association studies for personalized health care. Genomewide association studies are beginning to provide robust information for new genetic markers for common disorders. The research has been described as that which could lead to "molecular diagnosis"—enhanced tests for diagnosis and prognosis of disease. These studies may also have the potential to discover genetic markers and screen for disease. Although the application of genomic medicine seems futuristic, concerns have been raised regarding the ethical standards of tissue banks, the value of personal privacy in a network of market exchanges, and the protection of genetic information stored as inexhaustible computer data.

The new genetics of genomic medicine takes another shape by using association studies in pharmacogenetics and pharmacogenomics targeted at both patient populations and individualized variations. This development is intended to advance drug development technologies by investigating the role of disease-related genes in drug response. Several trials are already under way to examine the usefulness of testing for variants in genes for selecting drug therapy and dosage selection. Researchers have come to understand they are looking for variations in multiple loci in multiple gene systems. They have also come to understand that the relationship between gene and disease may show some consistency across populations, but that the relationship between gene and disease and drug shows much more variation. Once the multifactoral relationship between genes and disease is found, pharmacogenetic testing can be considered in order to prescribe the best possible drug. The magic-bullet drug becomes a real possibility. Rather than to develop a one-size-fits-all drug for mania and for use on the mass market, the goal would be to find new drugs that could be aimed at specific molecular targets for bipolar disorder.

Mania as a hereditary trait has traveled from an object on a pedigree chart to a "master control gene" to a genomewide associations and molecular diagnosis in personalized medicine. Eugenic psychiatry once marked a destined manic fate on the affected individuals in genealogical charts as blackened squares and circles to trace an inherited trait through generations. The rhetoric of a "gene-for" bipolar disorder in the search for "master control genes" in classical genetics transported the genetic marker to individuals.[28] Association studies across large populations of individuals hold a promise for molecular diagnosis of bipolar disorder in personalized medicine. This promise has come into being in new genomic medicine, but only in the verification by genetic testing that the genetic markers are really there. To achieve pharmacogenetics and pharmaco-genomics, individual genetic testing would have to be woven into the practices of drug therapy.

If achievable, molecular diagnosis in genomic medicine would pin down the objectness of mania. Is it significant, then, that these studies begin with madness? That they begin with what have been established as the performative symptoms of mania: thinking one has special powers, plans, talents, or abilities; engaging in sexual indiscretions or reckless driving; behaving in ways that are provocative, obnoxious, arrogant, or manipulative; having increased activity or excitement; experiencing delusions or paranoia? The symptoms of madness are translated into a bipolar diagnosis and travel, hanging on in a partial connection, to molecular genetics. If achievable, pharmacogenetics and pharmacogenomics will find the gene and disease and drug relationship so that drug therapy can be targeted in personalized health care. When pharmacogenetics and pharmaco-genomics begin with the identification of disease-related genes and develop the "drug-for" bipolar disorder, will mania hang on to mad symptoms in screening for successful diagnosis and drug response? If diagnostic identification and drug efficacy become possible, what will mania come to be if no longer the collective symptoms of madness?

CHAPTER 4

MANIC LIVES

MAD MEMOIRS

It's the first time I remember hearing the term manic depression, *and it sounds serious to me, conjuring up images of patients running around a mental ward half naked in terrycloth slippers—it sounds like the word* maniac.

—Andy Behrman, *Electroboy*

Mania has been recognized by physicians from the first century to the twenty-first century as both general madness and a form of madness with unique qualities. But no medical account can describe adequately what those who suffer mania experience. No description of mania in textbooks or asylum reports, and certainly not in genetic studies, measures up to the detail of firsthand accounts. Those who experience bipolar illness who write about their experiences are quite aware that they are symptomatic. Mental illness narratives have appeared in unprecedented numbers in the last decade, many of them in the form of bipolar autobiography. These writers know all too well the experience, not the theory, of writing as a storyteller with a pathological tale to tell.

Andy Behrman's memoir *Electroboy*, for instance, begins with an admission that there can be "a great deal of pleasure to mental illness."[1] He describes mania when it comes in episodes with familiar adjectives like "excitement" and "stimulation." His mania creates what he specifically expresses as dreamlike states "similar to Oz." He often confuses his manic episodes with his dreams—his senses overloaded and his head "cluttered with vibrant colors, wild images, bizarre thoughts, sharp details, secret codes, symbols, and foreign languages" (xix). Describing mania as "desperately trying to live life on a more passionate level," he recalls flying from Zurich to the Bahamas and back in three days, spending $25,000 on a shopping spree, and binging on alcohol, sex, and drugs. And so Behrman also points out that mania is "about blips and burps of madness" (xvii). It is delusional and irrational and out of control. It is buying twelve bottles of Heinz ketchup and eight bottles of Windex in the middle of a sleepless night or shoplifting a toothbrush and some Tylenol just for the high. Behrman is clear, however: "Pure mania is as close to death as I think I have ever come" (xix). He concludes his preface by emphasizing that the euphoric highs of mania were "out-of-control episodes that put my life in jeopardy." There is no creative spirit or love for life driving mania and there is no controlling the insanity: "actions are random—based on delusional thinking, warped intuition, and animal instinct" (xxi).

Memoirs like Behrman's offer alternatives to the celebrity testimonies about the dangers of mania. Indeed, actor Patty Duke and television journalist Jane Pauley, for example, have published their stories in an effort to increase public awareness of the experience of mania as one state on a bipolar spectrum and to reduce the stigma associated with bipolar disorder.[2] These memoirs offer hope for recovery and the experience of a return from illness to a kind of health. Unlike these celebrity memoirs, the memoirs considered throughout this chapter provide insight beyond the narrative identity of the celebrity. Rather than modeling the recovery or survival of a healthy and intact individual, these narratives offer another kind of credibility, detailing the always present chaos of the illness, a continuous threat without resolution.[3] Printed by small presses or self-published, the narratives are those of ordinary individuals with bipolar illness. The writers draw purposeful and playful attention to a loss or suppression of memory and write about delusions and hallucinations, and the consequent unreliability of narrative authority when there is no way out.

However, many literary theorists express skepticism regarding autopathography—that is, autobiography focused on or inspired by the influence of a disability, disease, or disorder on the author's life—especially as autobiography itself has come under suspicion in the twenty-first century. The (im)possibility of writing autobiography of any kind as an act of self-representation in a postmodern age after the "death of the author" has put the integrity of the narrator and the reliability of the narrative in question. Nevertheless, as a response to such criticism, which threatens to undermine the reliability of autobiography as a literary form, authors like Dave Eggers have treated narrative less as the normative translation of an individual's account of "what really happened" than as transgressive play with the trustworthiness of an author or the delivery a reliable narrative. Truth telling is often supplanted by the literary art of imaginative storytelling.[4] For some literary theorists and cultural critics, however, no imaginative storytelling can solve the complications of autopathography. When autopathography takes the form of a mental illness narrative, some critics argue that the lack of a coherent and continuous identity precludes an ability to recapture earlier selves, reinhabit former memories, or recover anything more than episodic narratives of unpredictable instability. The difference between autobiography and autopathography is one of purpose and intent—playful or pathological. The question raised for autobiography is, "How ought we read when any narrator breaks the contract with the reader purposefully, and intentionally flaunts conventions by crafting playful autobiography?" The looming question for autopathography is, "How ought we read when memory loss or other disabilities prevent performing self-narration according to the rules, or performing it at all?"[5]

Performing Not at All, or in More Than One Way?

The critical challenge regarding the performance of autobiography in mental illness narratives is whether these narrators can perform at all. Addressing this challenge means confronting the interrelated assumption that those living as subjects with mental illness cannot tell stories about their self-experience with mental disorder. Telling a story of mental illness requires using the language of diagnostic criteria, and this language "guarantees a kind of noncommunication." Mania can be told, if told at all, only in the language of mental illness—and this language does not communicate. Further, the language of madness is too garrulous, rambling, and effusive to perform a recognizable manic narrative. Madness is unspeakable in a space of "intense and ubiquitous verbalization."[6] We must be able to talk about mania in a discourse of mental illness and narrate mania as madness in a language describing a truly debilitating condition—"Can we have it both ways?"[7] In other words, can we trace the medical and linguistic constructions of mental illness and also imagine the reality of living with madness?

It is necessary to turn to a brief summary of Foucault's view regarding the question of whether the mad can speak, a question that informs the persistent doubt that madness can be performed in narration. According to Foucault's allegory, a shift in the idea of madness occurred when the mad stopped being treated as fools and started being treated as patients. This shift separated madness from reason—madness as tragic separated from mental illness as a diagnosis by a medical community. A central point for Foucault is that the split between madness and mental illness "affords a broken dialogue."[8] What remains is a monologue in which the language of psychiatry has been established, while madness has been silenced. The claim extracted from Foucault's literary and rhetorical approach to madness is a literal rather than a metaphorical one: we do not know how to speak about psychiatric disorders without reference to psychiatric medicine, and therefore we cannot speak of madness as anything other than mental illness. The claim assumes a rupture in the broken dialogue, a chasm that now exists between mania and madness.

In this book, madness continues to linger with mania as mania has become mental illness. Both madness and mental illness do speak, and when they do, they echo one another, allow us to think differently about embedded symptomology and embodied symptoms, and act recursively in ways that enlarge the interconnections between madness and mental illness. The language of mental illness is noncommunicative only if madness is not heard within in it. And madness is so ubiquitously verbose as to be unruly and inarticulate only if it is unaccompanied by mental illness. The narratives quoted in this chapter have been written by people who do not care to attend to theories of medicalization. They participate in a medical community by the very focus of their inquiry into their mania, but their descriptions of diagnosis are not necessarily noncommunicative. The most distinctive trait of these narratives is a convergence within the inquiry, an inclusion/exclusion of mental illness and madness. At key moments, these authors can speak madness, even if verbosely, and do so in ways that communicate something both within and outside of mental illness.

Is Authentic Narration of Mental Illness Possible?

The first challenge to mental illness narrative asks whether the discourse of mental illness can be narrated as a true debilitating condition. Here, questions of reliability take on additional layers in mental illness narratives, as the assumptions now are multidimensional: is it "the author" writing this story or is it the author's pathological or therapeutic identity or both? The assumption is that the author is only a constituted medical identity under the influence of the psychiatric classification of symptoms and the eventual effects of medications. Authors with mental illness—even (or especially) those treated with medication—can tell a story only as someone so radically altered by illness and its treatment as to make it impossible to fashion a reliable narrative, or to engage the reader in anything other than a fictional self-story.[9]

When Lizzie Simon completes her literary project, Detour, and her literal road trip, she admits that there is always a nagging question: "How much of me is me, and how much of me is this illness?" Simon's story begins when she is seventeen and proceeds, as she describes, in subplots. After difficult years of studying overseas, Simon graduates college and works at a radio station but is restless to find her clan, as she says—to meet other bipolars like her. Simon sets out to interview others of her age diagnosed with her illness. When she returns from her "detour," she looks back over her own experience to find answers to her own question, and she notes that her memory necessarily fails her, because "we are unreliable witnesses."[10] When Simon admits to experiencing a divided self, the reader must approach the narrator as someone negotiating multiplicity, creating a narrative that is always partial, as well as playful and intentional. Never, as Simon emphasizes, is it merely "gobbledygook." Here Simon approaches her narrative with respect for bodily experience that is grounded in language. And despite divided, multiple, or partial selves and thus stories, she writes knowing that speaking madness, and speaking of madness, gets work done.

Authors of mental illness narratives know all too well that accounts of mental illness of any kind are necessarily flawed. They deny the very possibility of authoritative accuracy by intentionally crafting blurred plots that attend explicitly to loss of memory and double identities. Mike Barnes, describing a "spiraling" mania in his narrative journey *The Lily Pond*, recalls writing when there was "little left of me to remember."[11] Even at the beginning of his memoir, as he chronicles it, "I was slipping by steady degrees out of my life" (11). He describes voices he hears—not external voices, but the internal ones we all hear. One of these voices, "heard still this side of madness, which though is heard and recognized internally, has something external, not us, and particularly authoritative about it" (100). Later he describes these things as coming on subtly, until he feels like a "deepening confusion" that is "not me, not my life" (144). When at the end of his book, he thinks about the beginning and first episodes of mania, he asks with a nagging doubt, "Could it [mania] be over?" (188). Writers of mental illness narratives assume their narratives are flawed as memoirs and do not attempt to prove otherwise. They themselves raise the question of their trustworthiness, many admitting to being suspect but asserting that they are no less credible at performing as a storyteller.

Behrman, whose words open this chapter, includes close to the end of the book transcriptions of journal-like entries composed over the course of a year that express despair at his paralysis as a result of living a life with an "intangible illness": he simply cannot, he says, "just grab the manic depression in my hands and smash it into pieces or burn or bury it."[12] These writers "muck about" as they are "practicing at loss" and telling the "story of grappling" as they attempt to craft narratives out of what are blurry distinctions between the vocabularies used to describe themselves and their symptoms, to talk about diagnosis and treatment while expressing their emotional states.[13] They perform multiply, detailing the real experience of mania, identifying the medical symptoms and treatments for a disordered body and brain, and attempting to articulate the embodiment of mania as they have felt, suffered, and endured it, all spilled forth from a somatic self.

By now, scholars understand that in the act of remembering, individuals make sense of their lives in relation to the lives of others—that all memory is collective and cultural. Narratives are told and retold, mediators of later narratives and mediated by those that came before: a "recycled reality."[14] Narrators of mental illness memoirs recognize this mediation—they associate their individual bipolar identity with their participation in a bipolar collective. This "recycled reality" is not lost on Simon, who by the end of her detour has realized that everyone diagnosed with bipolar disorder has similar symptoms: "Everyone has stories about being dangerously violent," and "everyone has stories of being reckless with shopping, or sex, or drugging," and "most of us have seen things, done things, made things, achieved things no regular person could do," and "everyone has had some horrible tragic events happen." Further, "everyone has stories about being misdiagnosed, mistreated, misunderstood, and disrespected by the medical community." Finally, she says, everybody she has met who has been diagnosed with bipolar disorder feels lucky to have survived an often fatal illness, "feels lucky to be alive."[15] And yet, she says, these are the public noises and not private responses. For Simon and the other authors of mental illness narratives included here, the public noise made by mania may be spoken with the language of mental illness, but the private noise of madness remains, making itself heard even within this language.

Every collective memory, every shared symptom, and every public noise that Simon lists can be heard in the private minds of individual embodied and disembodied experiences of mania. For example, Keith Alan Steadman, in *The Bipolar Expeditionist*, describes a "yo-yoing" mind and a first encounter with bipolar mania. He says that as his mania progressed, he danced and pranced around town and eventually saw "imaginary characters that were incubating deep within [his] crazed mind." He describes bipolar mania as "mind mayhem."[16] Holly Hollan, in her memoir *Soaring and Crashing*, describes a first vision, a first break with reality, as an adolescent and details her "bipolar adventure" throughout adulthood, depicting the "twilight zone" of mania. At times, "reality ceases to exist." While experiencing what she describes as a "TOTAL loss of identity," she also feels she has "touched infinity."[17] Marc Pollard, in his short narrative *In Small Doses*, recounts the "rollercoaster" ride someone with bipolar knows as a "normal experience." He too speaks of losing his "grip on reality."[18] And so throughout the book, Pollard describes the impossible attempt to interpret "normal" events as anything other than what they are: wonderfully, hopelessly, and irreverently manic. A girlfriend, a job, and a bank account are all lost to the "omnipotence of mania."[19] Here, mania is enacted in the mediated and thus multiple space of public and private loss, where mental illness and madness continue to mingle, where the language of mania is still linked to the communication of madness.

What might be identified as the predetermined symptomology of bipolar disorder takes on individual shape in the specific behaviors of individuals, and these, too, speak to the ways in which the narratives are never fully infused with mental illness but remain tinged with the noise of madness. Steadman, for example, describes his assumption that those watching his manic and "exhibitionist" behaviors were on his side, rooting for him, so that "picking germ ridden cigarette butts off the floor, then smoking them in full view of busy shoppers was perfectly alright." He runs from pillar to post looking like a lunatic after sniffing crazy glue, all the while assuming he has an audience of caregivers, not oglers.[20] Hollan breaks the medicalized silence by chronicling the sense that she will find a cure for cancer, that the ways in which she moves knickknacks around is of spiritual significance, and that her own universal language will solve all problems. She chronicles a long list of events that mark her episodes, for example, she "cannot stop spending money."[21] Pollard tells us not only that he lost a bank account, but that "in October 2000, [he] filed for bankruptcy."[22] John Forkasdi, in his memoir *The Secrets Within*, remembers "hearing voices" telling him to buy things. And when he heard the voices, he welcomed them. He describes walking into a Mazda dealership and on the spot trading in the family Camry for a racy two-seat convertible.[23] These descriptions mimic the textbook language of psychiatric symptoms only by detailing the practice of lived experience of the symptoms.

The symptomatic discourse of "grandiosity" or "hypersexuality" fails to grasp all the noise of multiple social worlds or all the psychosocial pain and suffering of one body that is never the same body. Donald Kern, providing testimony for his narrative *Mind Gone Awry*, fancies himself a guru receiving telepathic thoughts from a higher power instructing him to lead the world toward something holy.[24] He uses a general reference to medical symptoms when he says explicitly: "The hallmark of [his] mania is grandiosity." He emphasizes experiencing a "delusive reality" in which he felt he needed to have an impact on something bigger, something holy.[25] Forkasdi, recognizing that he is not making sense, also vaguely recalls believing he was a "supreme being." Christopher Palmer, who has written extensively on the subject of bipolar disorder, more specifically describes imagining that, as a writer, he is "in the same class as William Shakespeare himself."[26] Hypersexuality also appears as a generalized symptom. For example, Hollan refers generally to sexual indiscretions, a loss of any sense of propriety, one night of mistaken judgment, fumbling for zippers and then slithering out of a coworker's house. In a lived way, in *Manic: A Memoir*, Terri Cheney describes hypersexuality by recalling her former life as a high-stakes litigator. In mania, her body remembers that same tingling sensation and sweet exhilaration, now in tight jeans and transparent silk shirt. In one poignant detail she makes her point: "true mania never steps out the door in anything less provocative than spike heels or sling-backs." When talking about her many sexual encounters, she warns that there is a "fine line, indistinguishable at times, between charismatic and crazy."[27]

There are simply times, however, when the language of symptoms cannot be constrained by the bodily experience of "impulsivity." Palmer writes at length in *The River Manic* about impulsive behavior and the consequent shame when mania passes. He is emphatic when describing the danger of his manic impulsivity. He had broken the law by damaging personal property—"all of a sudden I was doing it and I could not help myself." This was, he says, "the single-most manic period of my life," and it ended in his "earliest confrontation with the law [which] would nearly destroy" him.[28] Kern, early in his book, says that delusions often lead to impulsive acts: disrobing in public, cursing at strangers, and having imaginary conversations with world politicians. When he was manic, he said, there was no way to avoid these kinds of acts.[29] Cheney talks not only about sexual impulses, but also about stronger impulsive desires "to strike out and break something, preferably something that would crash and tinkle into a thousand satisfying tiny pieces."[30]

Finally, narrators of mental illness must work at constructing consensual reality, rather than contractual truth, with readers by emphasizing access to meaningful language. This is true when Marya Hornbacher, an award-winning writer, describes the origins of her mania in a book she titled, simply, *Madness*, in what is perhaps the most terrifyingly detailed account of the devastation bipolar disorder can have on sufferers. She draws attention to the double existence in manic lives, cautiously making this observation: "You have no idea that your symptoms are symptoms; they seem like completely reasonable behavior to you."[31] She reads her own writing and admits: "When I read it over, it's like two different people are writing it" (49). At one point she describes herself as "possessed" and at another point she uses a familiar literary image: "I turn into Jekyll and Hyde" (74, 146). When Hornbacher addresses her manic identity explicitly at the end of her memoir, she tells the reader that whatever madness brings, it's mine: "I am who I am," and "both things are true" (275). And, she says, she can write the story. She insists that she'll "show them" that she's "a writer" and that she's "real" (39).

Alternatively, Mike Barnes, in *The Lily Pond*, admits that when writing about mania from the beginning to what will never be an end, "none of this seemed sayable." However, on the last page of his memoir, he has nevertheless turned back to writing.[32] The speaking never seems meaningless, whether entirely intelligible or not.

CAN THE MANIC COMMUNICATE AND THE MAD VERBALIZE?

The second critical challenge to mental illness narratives considers whether those who are mad, those with mental illness, can narrate at all. These narratives are so powerful because their authors meet a fairly arduous dual challenge: narrating the noncommunication of mental illness in the ubiquitous, verbose, and chaotic language of madness. Andy Behrman, in *Electroboy*, admits that he is "not able to articulate the intensity of what's going on inside [his] brain" and when he acknowledges that his behavior is out of control.[33] Behrman must be persistent in explaining the excesses of mania, not only feeling out of control but "enjoying every minute of this craziness" (97). For some critics, Behrman is performing a script of madness with muddled verbalizations. His experience is at once appropriated when he admits, "I have a mental illness" (230). His narrative has been "talked into being" by medicalized language and appropriated by bipolar disorder. Consequently, the criticism describes his as a script that communicates nothing of an embodied experience, merely an already constituted mental illness. And yet, Behrman can say of the time when he was told he is manic depressive: "The words torture me still" (251). It is significant that when Behrman describes his episodes in the discourse of mental illness, he also refers to fits of rage: "manic depression rages out of control" (240). For Behrman, mental illness does not silence madness, it rages with madness.

Cheney's reaction to the diagnosis of mental illness also confronts the noncommunication of mental illness by narrating with an acute rather than a ubiquitous verbosity. Once diagnosed with bipolar disorder, an author must grapple with the diagnosis but is limited by medicalized terms. Cheney provides a finely detailed description of one medical symptom of the illness in what might be described as the supposed noncommunication of mental illness: "The clinical term for this is 'pressured speech.'" And yet, she speaks back to this ostensible noncommunication, living with bipolar disorder within the terms of mental illness, by asserting with greater verbal intensity: "pressure-cooker speech is more like it."[34] She fills in this description with keen imagery: "The urge to talk gets greater and greater as you head up the mood scale, until finally it is as irresistible as a sneeze in a dust storm." Then she describes reconciling with a diagnosis: "It's chemical I told myself" (111). For Cheney, "the label mattered," for "it made sense of my erratic life" (161). She goes further, describing her diagnosis as "genuine insanity" because "it occupies a whole different space in the DSM-IV." And finally, she admits: "I believe in this diagnosis" (162). The coming-to-know of a diagnosis is narrated through what Cheney finds to be a wholly communicable medicalized discourse and an acute verbosity of the embodied feeling of her mania.

Nearly every narrator testifies on behalf of the reality of the bipolar diagnosis and the process of negotiating with madness. Melody Hope, in her memoir *In My Head*, describes a depression at twenty-two and a first mania at twenty-six. Of her first reaction to the mania, she recalls refusing to admit that she was bipolar and thinking that "needing a psychiatrist was unheard of unless you were crazy." In the very last line of the book, Hope admits: "I have bi-polar disorder."[35] Jane Thompson considered herself a normal person until age thirty-two, when she was first diagnosed with manic depression. She wrestled with the diagnosis, first refusing to believe that she had anything in common "with these people." Even after reconciling with her diagnosis, trusting doctors, and reading books, she says: "I tried my best to forget that I was bipolar."[36] Hollan begins to struggle with the question, "What is normalcy?" and first attempts to understand the diagnosis by describing herself as "manic, insane, and psychotic," as she was out of touch with reality. She makes sense of mania by showing fMRI images of manic brains, explaining the processing centers, and emphasizing how important it is to learn specifically "how to recognize the manifestations of primary symptoms brought on by chemistry." Because manic states cannot be controlled, she tells readers, the only remedy is the influence of medication.[37]

Hornbacher, in time, discusses her relief at having a label for her experience: bipolar. If what was happening to her "has a name, it's a real thing, not merely my imagination gone wild." She says outright, "I'm sick." And she knows it isn't going away; there is no final cure.[38] Kern also draws attention to the word "bipolar" and describes it as "a world determined by biochemistry gone awry."[39] He too recalls knowing something was wrong and feeling eventual relief with a diagnosis: "Manic depression—mentally disabled." Perhaps, he admits, there was "mild disbelief," but he had known that "something major had happened."

Disbelief gave way to a "desire to understand the illness."[40] Hope similarly describes knowing something was wrong but not knowing what it was: "I'm crazy, I thought, or do you really call it crazy? Do you call it insane, or do you call it a chemical imbalance, or did I have a behavioral problem?" Finally, she too is relieved that she "got the treatment and the medication" she needed.[41]

The narrative of diagnosis is never crafted in a way that completely ignores the sensations of feeling different, of living in a word shattered by madness. A diagnosis may, in the conventional terms of psychiatric classification and optimistic treatment, come as some relief. But there is always the looming breakthrough, the terror and the panic of a collapse. There is, as Barnes says, always the apprehension that "something is gaining on him."[42]

Fear of such a breach permeates the narratives in their discussions of medication. Steadman recalls the day he was "presented with the news" that he was "suffering from the grand title of manic depressive illness" and emphasizes: "It was imperative to achieve as soon as possible an acceptable level of lithium in my bloodstream."[43] Every narrator describes experiences with finding the right medication or combination of medications: lithium, Lamictal, Depakote. When discussing her relationship with medication in *Detour*, Simon notes that "mental illness interacts with the way you define yourself from the moment it enters your life."[44]

Mental illness interacts with one's body from the moment one starts taking medications. Many authors describe the "toxicity" of their medications, especially early in the trial phase. Thompson writes of the troubling side effect of lithium—her whole body shook. She mentions specifically her trembling hands, the trembling so severe she could not sign her name. And yet, much later, she describes another drug as working so well she would never stop taking it: "You wouldn't catch me going off my meds."[45] Certainly, narrators have learned the theories of various medications. Hollan coins her choice of medication as her "golden nugget," describing its work as "affecting the activity of some key brain chemicals."[46] She explains that when the activity of these chemicals is too high, her medication lowers them, and when too low, her medication raises them. The drug, she says, helps her avoid emotional crises. Before she found this particular drug, however, she sifted through other options with undesirable side effects that set in nearly as soon as the drugs entered her system. One drug made her so sleepy, she drove off the road; another made her legs swell "so badly the skin was stretched to the point of cracking and my lower appendages looked like they belonged to an elephant!"[47]

Of the daily struggle between her body and the medications, Hornbacher tells of starting the day "with a mouth full of pills" and then staggering around "with the onslaught of chemicals coursing through my brain, rerouting errant neurotransmitters, herding neurons into their proper rows, creating connections that need to be there and blocking reactions that don't." The description of problematic medications is coded by the revolt she imagines in her brain, yet her

sarcastic reading is only a modest resistance to her hope of keeping the possibility of change alive. Still waiting for medicine to find the right drug for her,
she looks ahead: "What if the madness wasn't always trying to speak through
my mouth, manipulate my emotions and perceptions, pull the levers like the
Wizard of Oz."[48] The promise of that therapeutic future, she says, makes her
almost dizzy.

In these mental illness narratives, descriptions of psychiatric classifications
and medicalized treatments are always linked to the bodily site—and verbalized
in ways that compel the language of madness. Mental illness speaks most elo-
quently through the language of madness. This way of reading the narratives is
so much more evocative than that of posing either/or questions regarding the
possibility of the noncommunication of mental illness or the garrulous speech of
madness. Hornbacher continues to struggle with her diagnosis, does not want
to admit she has mental illness. Suddenly "bipolar" is less a relief. It is a major
"mental illness—the psychos, the nut cases, the incurably insane, the muttering
bag ladies and bums, the freaks." She takes her meds because she wants to believe
that if she does "what they say" then she will not be one of the incurables and
"the madness will never bother me again."[49] The circulations are simply more
compelling when read as both/and—as both a pathology and a play, both mental and mad, both medicine and mood.

MIGHT MENTAL ILLNESS AND MADNESS SPEAK MULTIPLY?

The final challenge to narratives of mental illness is to speak of mania as being
multiple. Once again, I argue that mental illness and madness coexist, and yet
speak differently in more than one site. Between both mental illness and madness, mania multiplies in a seemingly endless coordination of medical practices
and bodily pains. I argue that the memoirs cited in this chapter demonstrate that
there is certainly a cyclic way of narrating bipolar: medical psychiatric diagnosis
(in circulating psychiatric and popular self-help texts) becomes both a welcome
conventional rhetoric and a means to describe the supposed unspeakable shock
and chaos of acute distress and chronic suffering (the real bodily experience of
mania). And yet the vocabularies of classification used to describe a bipolar disorder diagnosis remain fraught with aspects of the language of madness. These
narratives are recursive, collective, and cyclic in that they echo a contemporary
story of illness (including DSM, self-help, pharmacology, other memoir, etc.).
However, I assert that they are recursive in another sense. The stories are themselves recursive, because they echo the collective memory of madness, a rageful
fury, a vocabulary stretching back to antiquity.

My argument is that indeed the language of mental illness narratives mediates
the experience of madness. The language of mental illness is seldom if ever not a
part of the narrative testimony of madness. However, I claim that madness also
mediates the language of mental illness, shaping mental illness narratives and

memories of mania. There is an obviously interlocked encounter between medi-ated and lived experience. Mania is neither always already mediated nor entirely and completely lived. In this space, mania is uttered and written, coming to be, breaking apart, holding together, and taking shape.

The mental illness narratives considered in this chapter remind us that psy-chiatric discourse cannot adequately warn us just how perilous the journey through madness is. Steadman does warn us: "Manic depression is really just a collection of topical twists and turns in which a beginning cannot reach a rational conclusion" because "it never knows where to stop." Mania "drags the latest thought through the maze only to arrive at an illogical conclusion." It is, he says, "crafty, manipulative."[50] Mania leads to a life-threatening climax that "brings tears to more than one pair of eyes." It is "not knowing how one's mind will work day to day. It is gradually turning bonkers."[51] Pollard emphasizes the particular character of this madness as "warped, demented, even grotesque."[52]

Certainly, each memoir is mediated by all those that preceded it, and this interdependence informs the language of, and the description of, mad distress here. Simon is not alone when she uses medical language to describe herself as "sick." Neither is her narrative unique when she draws on a collective experience, feeling that something was wrong and saying: "And then I went insane." Finally, Simon draws purposefully not on medicalized discourse but on the language of madness when she pushes the limits of her expression: "I had been transformed into a raving lunatic."[53] Hollan also describes her experience in mania as a kind of madness when she says she even "looks wild" and describes her brain as "a savage beast." When manic, she is entrenched in a "deep, terrifying, mysterious, ominous, endless wilderness of mirrors."[54] Hornbacher too uses the language of madness to stress the increasing intensity of her mania, asking the familiar ques-tions: "What's wrong with me?" "Am I crazy?"[55] One day she can be calm, and the next day raging. It is like "flipping a switch" and then feeling an urge toward "ripping the bathroom sink off the wall" (56). "I feel like a Tasmanian devil," needing to tear and throw and pitch and rip. The madness "slides under my skin." She thinks: "I'm going nuts. I am nuts. I have always been nuts" (60). On being diagnosed, she is "crazy as a coot. Mad as a hatter" (67). Hope describes herself as an "uncontrollable maniac" with uncontrollable and bizarre behavior. Her "mind was broken."[56] Thompson is also intense in her description: "I was so manic I drove myself crazy," and "my life was spinning out of control."[57] Palmer repeatedly refers to moods that are out of control, a temper out of control, thoughts out of control. There was no controlling his mania. Forkasdi agrees that there is "no way to control it" and admits that "it's very scary after you come out of being manic to hear some of the things you did or said."[58]

Coming to be manic is itself a mad event, accompanied by confusion and questions. Suzy Johnston, who in *The Naked Birdwatcher* is even optimistic about her future and is able to come to terms with the fact that she "happens to have manic depression," begins by asking a question all these writers seem to ask

at some point: "Did this mean I was mad?"[59] Attempting to convince herself—
"I wasn't mad. I wasn't mad."—she says it was obvious even to herself that she
"was struggling to get a grip on an illness."[60] As Hope asks, "What was going to
happen to me?" After all, she recalls thinking, "I was not crazy, or was I?"[61]
When Forkasdi is diagnosed as having manic-depressive illness, he says, "the
first thing that came to my mind was that I was crazy," and, he adds, "I was also
scared."[62] Palmer too refers to fear, observing that he is "as scared of yesterday as
I am scared of today as I am scared of tomorrow."[63] Cheney articulates fear when
she asks the more than rhetorical question: "How could I be crazy?"[64] She
describes her madness as "the monster" and finds that "manic feelings are sometimes so brutally strong it seems like there is no way to endure them" (88, 97).
She warns that "manic depression is just too crazy for most people to identify
with, or have comforting platitudes for," because bipolar is "so out there,
beyond norm" (161). In her experience, "nothing's colder and lonelier than a
manic morning after" (100).

These aching minds and aching lives remind us that individuals diagnosed
as "manic" experience real madness. Without understanding the circularity
and collectivity of medical mental illness texts with mental illness narrative, we
silence both and are left in our own endless cycles of medical noncommunication. Judging mental illness memoir as inadequate, even dangerous, and finding
it "merely" recursive, a kind of silence in the ubiquity of verbose language, does
little to expand our understanding of the many senses of madness. The dialogue
between mental illness and madness does provide an opportunity to expand the
language with which we elect to understand these states and to bring mental
illness and madness into new kinds of being. This opportunity is available,
however, only if individual lived practices, medicalized communication, and
acute verbalization can make themselves heard, noisily, in multiple articulations
of madness.

SOMETHING IS WRONG

Throughout this chapter, I have argued that there is neither noncommunication
of mental illness nor a ubiquitous or mad verbosity. Medicalized discourses
and mad languages are necessarily collective, recursive, and cyclical. Narrators of
such illnesses must be willing and able to communicate—in a way in which willing and able can be understood only in the consensual reality the narrator enters
with readers. In this chapter, I am also entering a consensual reality by confronting the conventions and boundaries of autobiography and academia, as
I decide whether there is a kind of obligation on my part to participate in the
collective memory of mania. I am choosing to do so with peril, asking who will
benefit by my silence, what will come from my speech.

I don't know exactly when the indications that something was terribly wrong
started to show and then hang together so that I felt as though I were in trouble.

My parents could say more about the beginnings, but those are their memories and, even if collective now, I won't invade that privacy. Of course they thought my temper tantrums, even as early as age four or five, were a little extreme, as they marveled at the closet door left hanging on one hinge. By adolescence, my mother, I think, worried mostly about my drinking; she was the one who found the pill bottles filled with shots of liquor hidden in plain sight. My dad, I know, worried mostly that I was "boy crazy" and often picked me up early from the skating rink, phoned me at the pizza place, sought me out in hiding places on camping trips, or volunteered a bit too insistently on driving me to and from high school dances. Mom knew I had a hot temper. Dad knew I was dramatic and would sulk. They thought I was an extraordinarily difficult and stubborn adolescent girl.

My first vivid memory of a sign I might be mad is a memory of a blackbird that had died and been mowed over, chopped to black feathery and red bloody shreds, on the lawn of my college's square. No one took away the pieces. For four days I walked past a claw and a clump of feathers. Every day I wondered when the grounds would be cleared. I mentioned the bird to my then boyfriend, who drew for me what looked like an inkblot, thinking the artistic rendering would be comforting. At night I imagined the bird before I fell asleep, and I woke up thinking about it in the morning. I had awful dread at walking past where I knew it would still be, though tossed slightly by wind or torn a bit more by decay. One day I walked home and tried to kill myself. The college counseling center sent a priest to find me and drive me to a psychiatric clinic to determine whether I was a danger to myself or others. I packed, left school, and went home with my father.

I recall one of the last years of graduate school when I was working through my comprehensive examinations. At some point I realized I could feel my brain, and that I was feeling it crack. There were already fissures. I stayed up all night trying to find first words, then letters, with which to construct my essay. Suddenly, brilliance. All those cracks lit up—my computer screen flashed a glorious blue. I found the words and typed the letters—furiously, madly, and for hours. I turned the exam in. I knew it was either the most stunning piece of prose I'd ever produced or full of crazed thoughts, in which case I would fail, and that would be the end of it, all of it. I went home and took a bath—with bubbles and a bunch of pills, a manic suicide attempt.

What I remember between that exam in the fall and Memorial Day weekend is hard to say. Winter in Iowa dulls memory. But there must have been signs, and if I were trying to write a coherent narrative and construct a coherent identity, I might go back and attempt to reconstruct events during that time. Most of the moments have been pretty much forgotten. Maybe if I tried hard enough, but the activity in those months is elusive. However, those three weekend days confirmed for me that I was having more than just a difficult time of it.

If I recall enacting my symptomology, I would highlight the specifics of my outrageous spending. I was house-sitting for my closest friend, and I decided the guest room could use a good cleaning. Before I was finished I had bought blue paint, new linens in pastel pink, a chenille bedspread with matching pillows also in chenille, and three very large stuffed fish also covered with chenille in every pastel color. Accessories included lamps of various kinds so that the light would always be right. I spent all night painting and redecorating.

In the redecoration project, I used every credit card at my disposal. I bought amazing, framed Tamara de Lempika prints that to this day remain wrapped in my basement because they didn't match the color scheme. I bought a new stereo system with Bose speakers—because I knew Emmylou Harris was speaking to me and I needed to really hear her. More than three thousand dollars in less than three days. On the stipend of a graduate student. Then I put on a skirt and a pair of heels, applied more makeup than usual, spritzed on a bit of perfume, and headed for the coffee shop I hung out at every day. Instead, I ended up at the bar next door.

I keep the chenille bedspread in my guest room as a reminder that I was once mad enough to buy the thing. The chenille is discomforting. The narration of the mental illness and the living through the madness is discomforting. And yet, illness narratives in general, if they are to be successful in doing more than telling stories of pain and recovery, require some reflexive humor in the testimony. And certainly there is humor in madness—though I cannot necessarily see it when I relive this experience every month, sending my $565 payment to the bank that collected all my credit card debt.

The next week I called my doctor and explained that I thought something weird might be happening, maybe some reaction to the anti-anxiety prescription. I hadn't slept in days, I felt like my head was buzzing, I'd been pacing and shopping and drinking, and, well—I filled in the details about my weekend. She instructed me to come straight to her office immediately, not to stop anywhere along the way (do not pass go, do not spend another dollar). Now I was scared.

When I am manic, my brain is noisy, all static, alternating between high and low frequencies. Noise. I hear my neighbor's television, someone rustling through the garbage, cars in the street, branches in the trees, water dripping, doors opening and closing, the low hum of appliances on standby. I even see noise. Some noises are one-dimensional shapes—triangles or rectangles. Others are three-dimensional, mainly cones. The vibrations of the fence next-door look like cylinders. To hold off the noise inside my head, I create lots of noise of my own. I talk. I talk to anyone and everyone about anything and everything. Mostly, others describe me as magnetic and dynamic. Then, as my speech becomes more pressured, I notice that my students stare at me and my colleagues stare past me. The concept of time becomes profoundly strange. I am unable to concentrate on any one signal. I can't read, because I can't pin the words down. Certain words in particular become very loud and begin to radiate and superimpose upon others. The best I can do is stream above the text. I can't write, because words hurt. My vocabulary is unlocated and painful. Or I can't write because a few words are too present. I overuse repetition. I hate the sound of *t* but love *b* and *l*. I also love alliteration and am lulled into believing that my prose is alive, luscious, and multilayered.

I entered the dialogue with mental illness when I was first diagnosed with bipolar disorder and prescribed lithium. I was not keen on taking the lithium. I opted for therapy. Eventually, as symptoms persisted, I was treated at different times and in different places for anxiety and panic disorder, depression, and post-traumatic stress disorder. I was diagnosed with four different disorders by four different psychiatrists. I took Paxil, Wellbutrin, Remeron, Xanax, and Ativan. I was prescribed Depakote, Topamax, and Risperdal. None of it seemed to help.

I was a graduate student when I became certain something was really wrong. I needed to know more. So I sat in the Borders store in the middle of the psychology section and pulled books off the shelf. I remember skipping books on bipolar disorder because I knew that was a real mental illness and certainly I would not have a serious mental illness. That would be just too melodramatic— and I'd been known to be melodramatic. So I kept looking, thinking I'd stumble across something.

Then a title caught my eye: *The Unquiet Mind*, by Kay Redfield Jamison. I was thrilled at the find, thinking right away: "Yes. That's it. That's what I have. This might make sense." Except upon a closer look, this was a memoir about manic depression. Eventually, exhausted, I bought the manic-depression memoir and took it home. As I had expected, I thought as I read, "Now this woman is really crazy," and so "she is not me." And I am not crazy. Until I got to page seventy-five. Jamison was describing piles of credit card bills and likened "sifting through remnants of [her] fiscal irresponsibility" as an "archeological dig through earlier stages of one's mind."[65] She described her purchases: a stuffed fox and snakebite kits. She described unwrapped packages and unopened bags among the chaos of her home. She also described piles of writing, stacks of albums, and books strewn over her floors. It was starting to make scary sense. She described her behavior and her mind as "frenetic." Most importantly, she described herself as becoming "hopelessly out of control."

She is crazy. She is manic. Am I? I put down the memoir. Only later—after I finished my dissertation, rode my bicycle across Iowa, flew to ten different cities for ten different interviews, ended up in a tenure-track position in Rochester, New York, and started to feel like I should start decorating my new apartment in much brighter colors—did I go back to the first page of Jamison's book and read again. But I read differently this time. I read as though I were on an "archeological dig through earlier stages of one's mind."

Jamison talked about flirting with a dean at a faculty party. I remembered one of the first faculty parties I had attended. I turned a quiet lawn game into a drunken full-contact tackle sport. I didn't know then how safe this group of people was (and is), and how lucky I am. A few days after the party, I had the name of a good psychiatrist and had earned the title "tackle bocce queen." The title, for me, is synonymous with "tackle bocce maniac."

I am now forty-two, and twenty years from my first diagnosis. I take lithium. I also take Lamictal, Klonopin, and Lexapro. I continue to see my better-than-good psychiatrist, a brave and patient man who would describe my bipolar as "brittle" but always treat me as strong. Last week he said: "I'm afraid you see yourself as a bipolar freak—do you?"

Yes, in fact, that is exactly my point. I am bipolar and have a medical diagnosis. And I am a freak; I am mad. There are no two options; I am both and more. I can have it both ways. And, like the authors of the other narratives cited in this chapter, I can tell a good story.

Conclusion: Speaking of Mania

Certainly, my medical history is full of madness. And yet when I pose the question, What is mania? I am able to recognize my madness as no single manic illness. And so, the pressing question is not, Can the mad speak? but, What happens in the narratives of mania? How can we make meaningful sentences about the history of mania full of madness in the space in which mania and madness commingle?

The narratives here underscore the possibility and necessity of transcribing meaningful utterances into a collective, public memory of mania. Most of the narrators attempt to testify and to speak their mania to other bipolars. Hollan refers to a personal reason for writing about mania: so that other mothers will be able to recognize and understand their bipolar daughters. Simon, finishing her tour of herself, encourages others to go forward with their own investigations, to look back at first episodes for false memories and real memories and clues to recollection. Kern, who after struggling to survive is now helping others, wants to cultivate hope, but he also stresses the importance for him of remembering living with imagined historical figures and losing himself in a telepathic world. Remembering the shambles of one's bipolar past brings value to one's present life. However, these narratives are not relevant merely for the tangled memory objects included in them.

The simple assumption that there is nothing meaningful in autopathography is conceptually wrong. These mental illness narratives are relevant because they enact mania. Certainly, each individual expression and experience of mania has been mediated by the expressions of others—and those expressions mediated by yet others. Mediations can be traced in every direction but ought to be traced back to all previous utterances. Distinctions might be made between artificial or real utterances, or between the media in which the utterances appear. But the interdependence of these narratives must be fully accounted for if the history of mania and its multiplicities is not to be obscured.

CHAPTER 5

NEUROPSYCHIATRY, PHARMACOLOGY, AND IMAGING THE NEW MANIA

Could madness be seen in the living brain?
—Nikolas Rose, *The Politics of Life Itself*

If madness was medicalized in the nineteenth century—by the classification of mania as mental illness—it has been *technologized* in the twenty-first century by neuroimaging techniques and neuropharmaceutical entities that offer what may be more accurate means of diagnosing mental illness and discovering better treatment with more precise drug therapies. In the introduction to this book, I argued that a singular narrative of medicalization is too limited and limiting to account for the multiple ways in which madness gets made, unmade, and remade. One theme throughout my book is that there have been and continue to be different manias—not only different representations or different meanings, but multiple manias, more than one "real" mania. My argument has been that madness and mania are still very much coordinated objects, hanging together in a rhetorical history based on the layered practices of textbooks, asylum reports, genetic studies, and memoirs. Now, as we move into the neuro future, it remains to be seen whether madness will remain as tightly connected to mania.

This chapter examines the medical technologies by which mania is managed in neuroscientific research practices, discussing neuroimaging studies and the significance for neuropsychopharmacological application. The practices of neuroimaging and neuropharmacology are predicated on two interconnected promises, each of which premises cutting-edge access to the brain: (1) advancement in unraveling the real workings of the human mind/brain, especially the underpinnings of atypical brain activity; and (2) understanding of physiological states that will guide the invention of future therapeutic treatment. There is much here to create both discomfort and excitement: the move from working on cadaver brains to manipulating "live" brains, the methods of identifying atypical neural activity that has the potential to identify all brain abnormalities, and the potential implications for treating all pathophysiologically imaged human brains with purportedly precisely designed neuropharmaceuticals.

What has been declared the "century of the brain" has been greeted by many with energized optimism and predictions of a future in which complex interrelationships between human brains and medical technologies might redesign minds in hopeful, transcendent ways. Disorders might be aggressively targeted by psychopharmaceuticals and health optimized so that they become almost obsolete. If we believe that humans will become cyborgs or hybrids, it follows that our brains will be fundamentally redesigned as a merger between biological and nonbiological material, and neuroimaging will not provide the final or best scans of the visible brain.[1] Real-time, high-resolution, full-immersion images will be integrated into our daily lives. If mania can be seen in the living brain, it can be spoken of as atypical neural activity and treated more successfully with a specifically designed drug therapy.

Turning back, however, to the imaging technologies available presently, medical psychiatrists Roberto B. Sassi and Jair C. Soares, in their introduction to *Brain Imaging in Affective Disorders*, claim that neuroimaging technologies offer unparalleled advancement for studying mood disorders: "It is likely that in the near future these techniques will continue to develop at an even faster pace."[2] They describe the advancement as a "technological boom" that will help both identify the neural correlates of these disorders and bring to light the therapeutic actions of drugs currently used (or those that might be developed) to treat affective disorders. Researchers contributing to their volume echo this enthusiasm, describing these technologies as an "explosion" in advanced technology that allows greater ability to visualize the brain.[3] The attitude among all these researchers is best summarized as this: the time to invest in the intensive use of imaging "has now come."[4] Nancy Andreasen, a renowned neuroscientist and advocate of public understanding of how the brain works and of the developments for uncovering causes of mental illness, describes neuorimaging in *Brave New Brain* as a powerful new technology launching "a veritable voyage of exploration" that will identify deficits in specific brain regions and medications to both treat and reverse the illness.[5] The neuro future vision is one in which the brain and body mingle within a web of technology, constituting what it means to be human and eventually the transhuman.

Many writers have posited dire predictions for a neurological future, a "neurotransmitter revolution," expressing a fear that the neuron has been mistaken as the fundamental unit of the brain, and neurons firing as the production of all the functioning of our mental lives.[6] Here, some skeptics worry that research obtained from neuroimaging and potential image manipulations might have ominous political and ethical consequences. They predict the end of personal privacy as the result of neuroimaging techniques that will have the capacity to map brains, and a transfiguration of the human mind contaminated by psychopharmaceuticals. Not surprisingly, this fear has informed the popularized concern with both overdiagnosis and overtreatment of mental illness. For example, Peter R. Breggin, one of the more vocal skeptics, describes bipolar disorder diagnosis as once a rare case, a spectacle for physicians to observe while on rounds. Now, however, the diagnosis has become a "fad." According to Breggin, when mania is diagnosed correctly, it describes only "deeply disturbed persons."[7] Further, skeptics of neuropsychopharmacology ask whether treatment of behavior or personality has become a cultural phenomenon that results in the medication of perfectly normal people. Francis Fukuyama, for example, quotes extensively from Aldous Huxley's *Brave New World* to evoke the nightmares of science fiction, predicting the kind of political tyranny that could take place in a posthuman world in which individuals are no longer able to control their neurological makeup.[8] Fukuyama predicts that those organizing the neurorevolution will read minds to find madness everywhere, in any atypical activity, and will drug everyone. Without radical action, our human lives will become something darkly "posthuman."[9]

The fluctuation from the euphoric adoption of emerging technologies, specifically neuroimaging techniques, to the dystopic attitudes that regard these same technologies as grotesque tools threatening "the human" and the autonomous subject provides the background for my concern about the shape mania will take in our near future. The revolution threatens to alter humanity beyond recognition. If so, madness will have gone beyond mental; it will have gone neural, also altered beyond recognition. I agree that the exhilaration and optimism concerning new technologies may indeed be premature. The claims of seeing mania in the live brain are reductive. We do not see madness in the live brain. We don't really see mania. What we see is atypical brain activity interpreted as an indication of mania. And too, once such activity is located, its treatment will be identified, so the atypical brain activity is no longer visible as atypical. Mania will be overcome. I also argue that dystopic attitudes cling to a somewhat archaic notion of the human and an idealistic notion of autonomy. In what might be construed by some as a desirable postpsychiatry future, mania also disappears, no longer a faddish diagnosis. The diagnosis is returned to the truly mad or the "deeply disturbed." The mad, then, are left to their inhumane suffering.

I argue in this chapter that those who live the experience of mania simply cannot know with what reality we will live in a neuro future—but that despite an always underdetermined reality, we have to perform. And we will have to perform with the tensions created by neurotechnologies. The words and the discourses built around neuroscience in a neurotransmitter revolution have already created a space in which it seems likely that madness and mania may be enacted differently. Language about atypical neural activity may appear to put madness in tension with mania. Further, the imaging technologies may locate mania in the living brain and neuropsychopharmaceutics may then eradicate all symptoms of madness. Certainly, these symptoms would exist in other, more complex relations to each other. Mania may become less diffuse, more intensely real. Madness may pass away altogether. The purpose of this chapter is to determine what that transition means for the way the rhetoric of mania is handled—how it will be shaped, where it will travel, and how it will be manipulated in this transition. My questions in this chapter, then: Where will we see mania? How tenacious is the coherence between mania and madness and how will we know when the objects clash, separate, and come to be singular? Will we come to a new understanding of what it means to be human? And if so, will we have a new representation of "the maniac"?

Neuroimaging: Scanning Moods and Imaging Mania

The Clinical Neuropharmacology Research Center, associated with the National Institute of Mental Health, was established in the late 1950s out of a perceived need to investigate new drug development and evaluate the efficacy of new drug therapies. By the end of the twentieth century, basic neuroscience began using techniques for neuroimaging, claiming to provide what research psychiatrists deemed major breakthroughs in understanding that led to the identification *and* the treatment of psychiatric disorders. Because mood disorders may indeed be the most severe and life threatening, yet the least understood, of mental disorders, neuroscientists have staked a particular interest in studying the neural bases of emotion. In *Brain Imaging in Affective Disorders,* a text dedicated specifically to the neuroimaging of mood disorders, an estimate suggests that by 2020 the affective disorders will be a major cause of disability and the second leading cause of death worldwide.[10] The expressed belief is that new imaging technologies will provide important insight into the cause of bipolar disorder and the available treatment options, including magnetic stimulation, as well as traditional or inventive psychopharmaceuticals.

Neuroimaging technologies, like most medical research technologies, come together in bits and pieces, collaborations and competitions, with research and funding from academic and industrial sources.[11] These technologies—the CT scanner, the MRI (and fMRI), and the PET (SPET)—have all been sold on the concept that they can provide pictures of the wonder of the human brain. The technologies have been said to "see the brain at work" or "image the living brain" and even "see inside the brain" and track it as it thinks, regulates mood, and controls inhibitory mechanisms. A neurological approach to affective disorders, including manic depression or bipolar disorder, attempts to study the marker or cause of the mood disorder. Studies are inconclusive but suggestive, and different studies identify different markers: decreased paralimbic seratonin 5-HT$_{1A}$ receptors, decreased prefrontal phosphomonoesters, and increased basal ganglia chlorine. It would be tempting to pretend that we are now really seeing mania, that it is really there. If we see mania located in a slice of the brain, we will see a singular object and one disconnected from its madness. The tension between mania and madness may come finally to be resolved, and mania made solidly visible. However, this tension has never been neatly resolved. Not even the most powerful medical imaging technologies will handle the coordination so adeptly.

The CT (computerized topographic) scans are structural imaging technologies able to identify physical variations in the brain, such as ventricular enlargement and cortical atrophy, in what are thought to be severe psychiatric pathologies like mania. The CT scanner was the first brain-imaging technology to be presented as a machine that could see the brain. The machine did not, of course, allow the radiologist to see the human brain. The CT scanners did not even take a picture of the brain in the same way an X-ray "takes a picture" of the skull. CT scanners send out thousands of beams that intersect the brain at different angles; the data from those beams are fed into a computer to create a three-dimensional scan of the entire brain and eventually are made "legible," to be printed as a scan. After mathematical reconstruction and some enhancement, the computer produces an array of calculations that build the final picture.

MRI (magnetic resolution imaging) set a new standard for image resolution in structural imaging. Its developmental history is a complicated one, including contributions from chemists, physicists, engineers, mathematicians, physicians, and others across disciplines. MRI scanners magnetize hydrogen atoms in the brain. When these atoms become excited, their resonance can be detected. Atoms that are more excited produce stronger signals. Data collected during the course of imaging are processed with complicated statistical analysis and computer algorithms, which produce highly detailed, three-dimensional images. MRI can scan for markers of atypical brain structures, like lesions or signs of degeneration in the frontal lobe, potential indicators of a bipolar disorder condition.

The fMRI and PET are functional neuroimaging technologies that allow the neuropsychiatrist to look at the brain as it is functioning, to capture the processes of the brain. fMRI has been used extensively to study emotion, or mood states, in the brain. Functional imaging activates a region of the brain. When a region of the brain is activated, blood flow and volume increase and the supply of oxygen to the region is greater. The result is an increase in the oxygenated hemoglobin in regions of neural activity, perhaps indicating something relevant about the underlying etiology of mood disorder. For example, scans for functional atypicalities may mark an event like the blunting of what is expected to be an increase in activity at the left anterior cingulate.

PET (positron emission tomography) extended the possibilities for functional neuroimaging by examining molecular and chemical aspects of the brain. It studies cerebral blood flow. While PET revolutionized imaging technologies, it has its limitations—use of radiation, maintenance of the tool, and initial high cost. SPECT (single-photon emission computed tomography) is a strong imaging tool and is significantly more cost effective. Research using images produced by both PET and SPET may indicate dysregulation of emotion. By looking at blood and oxygen flow, these images indicate atypical aspects of neurotransmission.

The various imaging technologies provide different images of the brain, identifying different possible markers indicating different atypical brain anatomy or activity. We are, of course, not seeing mania, but markers that indicate mania. Further, any of these markers are just that—indications of something that must be interpreted. One marker might be overactive cortisol production in the hypothalamus region of the brain, which may not be providing the normal regulatory mechanism for this production.[12] But "watching" the brain produce too much cortisol is by no means "seeing" mania. Rather, the overactive cortisol production may lead to symptoms like insomnia, a suspected trigger for mania. When imaging techniques craft an image, what we really see are the markers—lesions, increased blood flow, and so on—taken to indicate atypical, perhaps manic, brain activity. In all of these imaging techniques, in order to identify the marker, data about blood or oxygen flow, for example, is collected and fed into a computer, where algorithms produce data sets. These data sets, a bunch of numbers, are substituted for pictures, images of the brain. All these techniques, markers, indications, and data sets must come together, must coordinate, for mania to come to be here. The technologization of mania in neuroimaging research will not necessarily make it a stronger object. Mania might as easily fracture into many bits.

Studies that use neuroimaging technologies are currently not diagnostic but research based, and so the studies begin by identifying a control group and a population already diagnosed with bipolar disorder. As such, imaging studies begin with preexisting enactment of manic symptoms and produce images that "fit" those enactments. Some studies begin with the familiar definitions of mania, here from a published report by Lori Altshuler: "In addition to an alteration in mood, the clinical state of mania comprises a cluster of symptoms involving increased impulsivity (e.g. overspending, hypersexual behavior, increased risk-taking behavior), impaired attention (distractibility), and increased motor activity (e.g., increased movement, increased talkativeness)."[13] Altshuler's study assumes that this cluster of symptoms indicates potential impairment of brain inhibitory mechanisms, and so focuses specifically on a region of the brain that might contribute to the impairment. The study speculates that decreased activation in the orbitofrontal cortex is associated with mania and disinhibition, but also with aggressive behavioral responses. Another study also begins with impairment but focuses on memory as one of many cognitive functions affected by pathological mania. This research of the cingulated cortex of the brain suggested anomalies in manic subjects.[14] Other studies also begin with particular manic symptoms like violence and aggression or dysfunction and disability. One of these cites "classic manic symptoms" as outlined in the DSM-IV, including "excessive maladaptive behaviors."[15] Another begins with the APA definition of mania, including irritability, distractibility, and impulsivity, and extrapolates the dangerous effects of mania in personal and professional lives.[16] All the studies begin with bipolar disorder and are thus studying not the brain per se, but symptoms attributed to mania already implicated in the brain. And so as mania enters the neuro future, it continues to sustain connections with madness across its rhetorical histories.

The very process of designing and carrying out imaging studies poses the question of *multiplicity*. Meta-analysis research points out the extent of variation across the results of imaging studies produced by different institutions and different studies. In imaging studies, there are competing approaches to the use of algorithms used to create data sets. The use of different technologies produces scans with significantly different resolutions. In addition, different scanners collect data over different time slices, with shorter peaks and valleys over brain activity. The multiplicity of results in imaging studies has much to do with the study designs, variation in technologies, and statistical analysis. Because of such differences, every study includes in its methods section the imaging procedure, the specific scanner used, and the software used for statistical analysis. For example, one study documents not only that an MRI machine was used, but specifically what type: a 3-T instrument obtained from General Electric in Waukasa, Wisconsin.[17] These studies also state how statistical information was obtained: data were processed with BioImage Suite, for example, or with Statistical Parametric Mapping software.[18] All this difference created by different techniques means that reality is still multiplying. The real mania is still a multiple reality.

The language used in the conclusions of imaging studies, in descriptions of the underlying mechanisms for the classical symptoms, may not be that of classical madness, but it does refer to mania as a brain abnormality or dysfunction, or as a malfunction. The results also follow the mechanisms of mania as they travel from one site to another, or from one region of the brain to another. Researchers argue that current studies point to multiple causes for bipolar disorder, citing the contributions of the corpus callosum, its subregions, and the corticolimbic network. Others cite an emerging picture that indicates the orbitofrontal lobe plays a role in bipolar disorder. Studies argue that the diversity of clinical symptoms suggests that affective disorders are a composite of functions of the extended limbic system and its neural circuitry. In examining the interconnected limbic pathways and neocortical circuits, it is also apparent that no single neurotransmitter abnormality can explain affective disorders. Any cause is "multifactoral."[19] The multiple technologies will not produce a unified mania, or one without a pathological performance or malfunction.

When imaging studies begin by looking for dysregulation of emotion and find the region of interest in the brain that is compromised, mania is once again stretched in two directions. It remains enacted as madness and pulled toward the language of the neurological. I argue that there is certainly some necessary, even if yet to be determined, physical connection between the manic brain as it has come into being as symptoms in a body, and the manic brain at the real, neurological level. My argument is that these imaging techniques cannot deliver the "real" mania by seeing its structure or its functioning in some region of the brain. Certainly, these practices actively bring mania into another kind of embodiment. They create a mania that is fragmented, sliced, and cut into pieces, and also enact a mania that remarkably coheres as a collection of mad bodies, multifactoral causes, and different data sets. Imaging technologies coordinate multiple ontologies, a different manic neurocircuitry and an indicated manic pathophysiology. When mania is performing in these scans, it is performing multiply.

How enticing to imagine peering into the brain and finding mania. And how easy to forget the difference, or lack thereof, between a coded scan and a similarly mediated picture. Medical imaging technologies of all types conjure the thing itself, as if it is right there. And we imagine that there finally is mania: coherent, coordinated, a single object. How easy to forget the multiple manias that appear in the multiple scans, none the same and always more than one mania in one scan. How easy to forget the multiple algorithms that make up mania. What if we also saw the numbers that make the technologies work? Something like $y = (1 - 2e-t/\tau)$ or $\mathrm{Sin}(\theta_1)\,\mathrm{Sin}(\theta_2) = 1/2\,\mathrm{Cos}(\theta_1 - \theta_2) - 1/2\,\mathrm{Cos}(\theta_1 + \theta_2)$. Or an equation for imaging manic brains that read something like $[F(1,71) = 11.2, p = .001]$ with FA lower in the middle CC ($P_{bonf} < .001$)? Would our gaze be quite so scopic or our desire to find mania quite so tactile? In early neuroimaging technologies, the worry among radiologists was that there were not enough numbers and that these numbers could not render useable scans. Now the numbers are hidden and those of us looking at the pictures that have moved out of the lab are mesmerized by compelling, colorful images. We do not ask, Who makes up the algorithms? Where do the exponential functions, differential and integrals, vectors, matrices, and convolutions come from? The numbers have scattered, lost in a conflict with the rich and intricate images. And yet the digits are no less an enactment of mania and not necessarily a sign of incommensurability between one mania or another.

However, the images themselves, the scans as highly mediated image analyses, have created curiosity as well as anxiety. Concerned with the presentation of the images as well as their visual rhetorical power, Joseph Dumit articulates a number of questions about how these brain scans will be used to create identities, most directly, "What if they are true?" Dumit has explored both the ways that neuroimaging works and what brain scans do in practice, and admits to both fascination and horror as he contemplates whether this technology will tell him who he really is. Dumit worries that neuroscientific researchers "share the *Idea* that the brain must be in some fundamental way the person."[20] There may be very good reasons for anxiety regarding the seeming fetishization of brain scans, the technologies, and their uses. Brain scans seem to persuade by

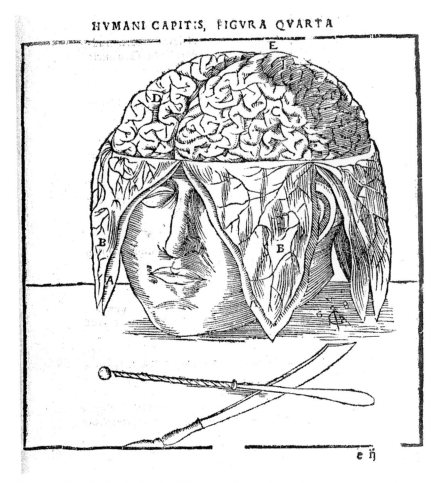

Figure 5.1. "The Brain: the Cerebral Cortex," Johannes Dryander, 1537. *Reproduced by permission from Wellcome Library, London.*

eliciting a phenomenological response. What, then, does a brain scan labeled "mania" really mean?

Of course, we have always been interested in images of the brain. And we have always pictured mania, whether through anatomy (figure 5.1), our advanced MRI scans (figure 5.2), or representations of the maniac in illustrations (figure 5.3) or in photography (figure 5.4). I am inclined to wonder here whether the brain scans labeled by the determined illness—mania—conjure up early fascination with illustrations of the brain as a particularly interesting organ, later nineteenth-century illustrations as spectacles of madness, and then medical photography of manic bodies. The illustration of the brain from the sixteenth century (figure 5.1) depicts the brain's cerebral cortex in a static sketch and, notably, includes in the medical instruments that would have been used to slice

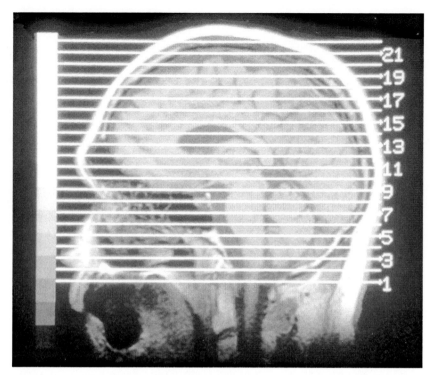

Figure 5.2. "Head and Brain of Adult Human Head, MRI." *G. Dimijian MD/Photo Researchers.*

a postmortem brain, providing the viewer with the imagined procedure. The sketch, which appears in an authoritative medical textbook, credibly labels parts of the brain's anatomy. The language of brain functioning in the twenty-first century is of functional, structural, and chemical abnormalities detailed in three-dimensional maps of real-time brain activity—those practicing with neuroimaging technology argue that an understanding of the human brain necessitates the ability to see the brain working "live" or "in vivo." The brain scan offers this real image (figure 5.2). Rather than an illustration, the brain scan offers an assemblage of slices of a live brain. However, neither in illustration nor in scan is it possible to find mania. There is no single brain specimen or single brain scan of the maniac that has become iconographic.

It is possible, however, to locate the icon of "the maniac" in photography. Esquirol's illustration captioned, simply "Straitjacket," depicts a man with wild hair and wide eyes, the jacket around his waist, and arms. His hands, not in view, are obviously struggling against his restraint (figure 5.3). In the photograph reproduced as figure 5.4, the images are iconographic of "the maniac." The hair is disheveled, the eyes wild, the mouth contorted. These bodies were frequently illustrated and photographed in the nineteenth and early twentieth centuries,

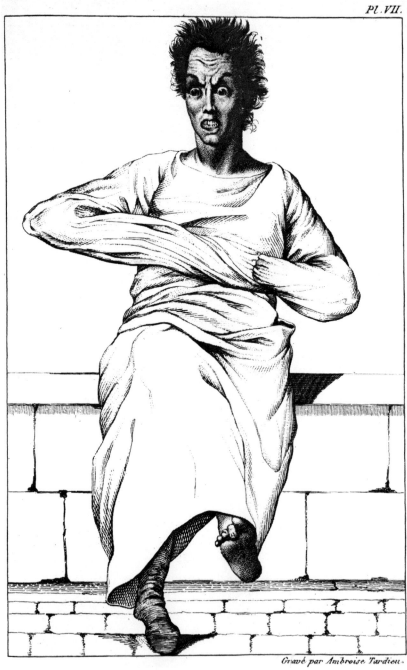

Pl. VII.

Gravé par Ambroise Tardieu.

Figure 5.3. "Straitjacket," 1838. *Mary Evans/Photo Researchers.*

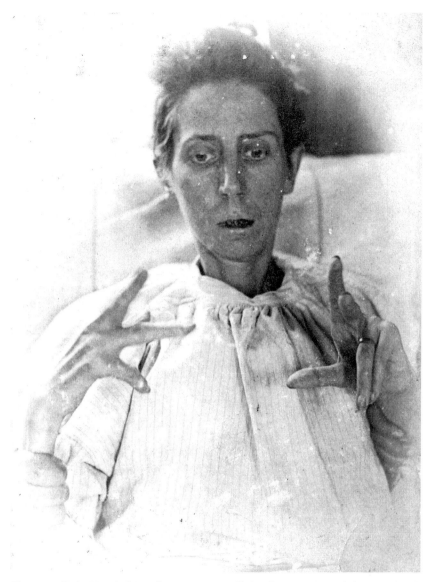

Figure 5.4. "Frier Hospital, London: a woman suffering from mania, with forearm, hand and finger movements. Photograph, 1890/1910," 1890. *Reproduced by permission from Wellcome Library, London.*

particularly in textbooks (see chapter 1). The physical appearances in these pictures from the nineteenth century are so similar as to represent mania as one category of insanity.

Today, the illustrative and photographic icon has been interrupted by a multitude of brain scans. In the scans, there are images from different angles, images that show different slices of the brain. As one stares at the radiant blue and red colors of what hardly looks like a human brain in a textbook SPECT image, captions inform one that these colors indicate patchy uptake throughout the cortex of a manic brain. The caption of an MRI image, gray scale, with pretty bright yellow spots, identifies a reduction in the volume of gray matter in prefrontal and temporal regions of the brain in bipolar patients. In a third scan, an fMRI shows the manic brain functioning in a cognitive task. The images again are gray scale, now with a spectrum of colors from yellow to orange to red, and the differences in color and distribution of color indicate a lower inhibitory control. These provide connections, but no a singular image of the maniac.

There are scans that show brain regions and others that show brain functions. And there are images using coloration from red and blue to yellow and red, as well as green, purple, and orange. It is important to recognize that all of these scans are spreading, multiplying in different ways. There have always been different versions of mania, and these have existed side by side, with and without friction. Neuroimaging does not give us an iconic "mania" and cannot develop "true" or "real" images, only mania by multiplication. The real feat of our imaginations is that the simple illustration and the analog photograph cohere with digital imaging scans under the label "mania."

PSYCHOPHARMACOLOGY: MEDICATING MADNESS/MADLY MEDICATING

Neuropsychopharmacology is defined simply as "the study of drugs that affect the nervous system."[21] Many neuropharmacologists have argued that it may be possible to use the knowledge provided by neuroimaging techniques to work with drug treatments more accurately. If neuroimaging aims to monitor the "in vivo" brain, the latest in neuropharmacology aims to monitor the "in vivo" brain once drug compounds have been administered. Neuropsychopharmacology emerged fully as a new field in the 1950s and 1960s. It was in the 1950s that discovery of medications other than the major tranquilizers occurred. The antidepressants classified as tricylic antidepressants (TCA) and monoamine oxidase inhibitors (MAOI) were made available throughout the 1970s and 80s. Additional significant work in the 1980s produced the serotonin reuptake inhibitors (SRIs), atypical antipsychotics, and mood stabilizers. Lithium for the use of its antimanic effect was an early discovery during these years of a new pharmacology, and it is still considered the "golden standard" for treatment of bipolar disorder. Yet lithium has always been a problematic drug, a particularly stigmatizing medication.

Lithium was discovered in 1817 by John Arfwedson and appears on the elemental table, following hydrogen and helium. It is the third-simplest element and the first solid one. The element was first used for medicinal purposes in 1843 and continued to be used in mineral spring water as a cure for various ills until 1898, when it was deemed "toxic" and taken off the market. A modern history might begin with John Cade, who conducted a clinical trial of lithium with ten manic patients and noted that the symptoms of mania disappeared—the first trial of lithium for its antimanic effects. Cade published a paper in 1949 documenting his conclusion that the lithium treatment was effective.[22] Studies by Morgen Schou confirmed Cade's initial result that lithium was therapeutic for patients with mania. Until the 1970s, however, without advocacy from the pharmaceutical industry, lithium lost its popularity.

Nathan Kline was influential in generating interest in lithium, despite the lack of backing by any pharmaceutical company—because lithium is a natural element, it had no commercial value. Kline pushed the American College of Neuropsychopharmacology to register for a new drug application. He worried: "There were cries that no American pharmaceutical company would produce the drug because it could not be patented and there would not be any appreciable profit margin."[23] Eventually two companies—Smith-Kline and French and Pfizer—applied to the FDA and received approval in the 1970s. Kline remained confident that investigations of lithium would lead to both a better understanding of mania and insight into its management.

It was also in the 1970s that Peter Breggin, a strong critic of neuropsychopharmacology, first described the relationships among pharmaceutical companies, academic researchers, the American Psychiatric Association, the Food and Drug Administration, the National Institute of Mental Health, and community lobby groups as a "psychopharmaceutical complex."[24] Breggin argued that the use of pharmaceuticals to treat the biological model of mental illness is "medical spellbinding" and ultimately damaging to the brain. He compares the use of drugs, or what he referred to as "medication madness," to the use of lobotomy and electroshock therapy (1). In the 2008 revised edition of *Brain-Disabling Treatments in Psychiatry: Drugs, Electroshock, and the Psychopharmaceutical Complex*, Breggin uses a scare tactic: drugs can be used to exert "every kind of authoritarian or totalitarian" control on human behavior (30). Breggin is not only a critic of drug therapy, however, but also a proponent of drug-free alternatives, including "moral therapy" of the kind proposed in nineteenth-century asylums as "humane" treatment without violent restraints. As an example, Breggin summons Samuel Tuke's 1813 treatise, citing a passage about violent cases of mania, and argues according to Tuke's philosophy that even the most insane patients possess some control over their moral and intellectual faculties. According to Breggin, Tuke's treatise is "as pertinent today" as it was in the nineteenth century (433). The drug-free alternatives echo nineteenth-century principles of moral therapy, among them, promoting a caring relationship, creating a utopian environment in which limits are established, maintaining always a respectful tone even when confronting hostile behavior, and calling attention to odd behavior so persons can take responsibility for their conduct. Breggin believes that even "deeply disturbed" people, even those with manic episodes, can be helped without medication if they decide to put themselves under the guidance of a doctor who is dedicated to these principles of moral therapy (457).

This radically pessimistic view of pharmaceuticals is expressed primarily by those who adopt Breggin's concept of the pharmaceutical complex and extend its reach. For example, Brian Kean describes a society of "mass medication" that would mean the erasure of human rights by "the essence of modern evil."[25] The arguments regarding drug therapy for all mental illness are part of a longstanding professional debate played out in nearly any bookstore: Peter Kramer's *Listening to Prozac* will be found near David Healy's *Let Them Eat Prozac*, and these will be shelved among works such as Samuel Barondes's *Better Than Prozac: Creating the Next Generation of Psychiatric Drugs*. Arguments have also noted the power of pharmaceutical companies, the problems of clinical trials, and the potential coercion that takes place when patients are prescribed medications they are told they need without being provided adequate information or giving full consent. Pharmaceutical companies have been vilified as colonizers, profit mongers, and totalitarians who have constructed a thoroughly pharma culture.

Given the standard story of the rise of pharmacology, the treatment of mania with lithium does not entirely fit the larger narrative of either market and profit or totalitarian capability, because lithium has followed an entirely different trajectory. Lithium treatment for mania, as Healy notes, was introduced and developed differently from other pharmaceuticals: "The origin of the modern use of lithium in psychiatry in contrast to the almost rational engineering of chlorpromazine has the qualities of a fable. It is a story involving isolated investigators, in out-of-the-way locations, with a sprinkling of extraordinary ironies, taking on and subverting one of the most stunning breakthroughs in modern medicine."[26] Lithium's long history in various medicinal uses, its lack of classification in the major drug categories (not an antidepressant or an antipsychotic or other), and its development outside pharmaceutical companies muddles the standard arguments regarding the patenting and marketing of the drug in any pharmacological marketplace. Its history thus also muddles any standard narrative of medicalization that could be told about mania. If the pharmaceutical history of lithium doesn't quite fit into the portrait of a "pharmaceutical complex" that treats mental illness with medications invented as mechanisms of social control, mania doesn't quite fit the narrative of medicalization that incorporates such a portrait.

Nevertheless, lithium's status as the golden standard for treatment of mania and its special effectiveness in preventing suicide set the drug up as a kind of pharmaceutical wonder. Further, its effectiveness specifically for the treatment of bipolar disorder (its lack of effectiveness for treating any other disorder) and its mythological "direct target" for treating the mechanism of bipolar disorder bestowed on lithium a significance not given to any other psychopharmaceutical. Lithium has never been a so-called designer or cosmetic or lifestyle or me-too or happy-pill drug, as Prozac and other popular medications have been labeled. It is generic and has no commercial value. Lithium has certainly been a target for critics of psychopharmaceuticals who want to point out its high levels of toxicity and low levels of patient compliance. The mode by which lithium works has not been well understood and so until recently, this drug lacked a potential biomedical explanation. Other classes of drugs could describe chemicals that worked, for example, by restoring serotonin and dopamine balance. Lithium had no such story. It worked because it worked. But it worked to do what other medications could not. Lithium managed mania. The very specific connection between lithium and mania in the history of psychopharmacology sustained mania as the multiple object it had come to be, mad and medical both. Mad in that mania required its own special, mysterious, and even toxic drug; medical in that it did seem to respond to this singular medication.

Many of us who experience true mania might interpret the effects of lithium differently, as a drug of choice that allows us to work without flight of ideas, to interact with others without pressured speech, and to act without dangerous spontaneity. Others of us would prefer living with mania and its highs. We all perform mania in different ways, and we all have different molecular makeups, so we come to medication in more than one way. Lithium has been described as a disabling drug that changes personality: the mythical crushing of some unique creativity, the grim absence of some inherent sparkling essence, and the fated loss of a special kind of luminous spirit. The "flattening" effect that some people experience has been well documented—though whether this flattening is a fading of manic symptoms or a depression of mood is debatable.

Resistance to the drug points to the dampening of manic elation, the potentially toxic side effects, and the stigma that connects lithium to mania. The drug is widely known to be toxic in large doses and can be damaging to the thyroid and kidneys. This toxicity proves to be unacceptable to many. Because lithium can be toxic, those who choose to take it must have regular blood tests to monitor lithium levels. Finally, because lithium is considered to be a drug specific to the treatment of mania and is not classified under any drug category or used for the treatment of any other illness, it carries a stigma that other medications do not. When a prescription for lithium is given to a pharmacist, so is a single diagnosis. The bipolar diagnosis is always visible in the prescription and then on the bottle. If, while in line to pick up the prescription, the word "lithium" is spoken out loud ("Hermsen, lithium?" and "Do you have any questions about your lithium prescription today?"), there is nothing but bipolar that can account for that word. While most psychopharmaceuticals treat more than one disorder, from anxiety to mild depression, lithium treats only one, and it is one that carries a different kind of stigma.

While neuropharmacology has provided significant evidence regarding lithium's mechanism of action, explanations of its efficacy remain elusive. Lithium in its early use had mysterious clinical efficacy. Its reputation paled in comparison to the wildly popular and less stigmatized minor tranquilizers. In the early 1970s Valium was the most prescribed drug in the United States, used for a vast array of ailments, for example, in sports medicine as a muscle relaxer.[27] By the end of the 1970s and through the 1980s, as Valium fell out of favor, Prozac replaced it as the new wonder drug, receiving commercial play from *Time* to *Cosmopolitan* as a white-collar drug popular with supermoms and business-people alike. In middle-class society, these were drugs not for the mad, but for the so-called working well who wanted to feel better than good.

Although the neuropsychology of lithium had not been understood in 1970s when the FDA approved it, once made available, lithium treatment for acute mania became a standard prescription for bipolar disorder. A 1969 three-part series in the *New England Journal of Medicine*, "Neuropsychopharmacology and the Affective Disorders," noted that the drug's effectiveness for treating the affective disorders had been important, as well, for psychiatry in general. Mention of lithium salts argues that this treatment must be distinguished from the antidepressants like Prozac, and notes the documented effectiveness for mania only.[28] The third part in the series hypothesized that lithium may affect norepinephrine and serotonin metabolism in the brain.[29] Lithium first became a stimulus for other neuropsychopharmacological research because, as a single natural element, it produces complex and unique neurological change. Lithium is not chemically produced, and it is the only drug that manages mania, and so it was thought to have some special properties.

Despite lithium's reputation as toxic, studies now find the drug of interest for its protective qualities. Indeed, lithium has become a valuable agent of investigation in neuropsychopharmacology, increasingly *for* the theories of its mode of action. Research into the pathophysiology of mania and other affective disorders suspects focal lesions in specific brain regions, dysfunction in neural pathways, and some implication of neurochemical systems. Studies have indicated some regional reductions in brain volume, especially in the hippocampus, which may be more susceptible to atrophy. And preliminary studies suggest there may be a progressive element to the disorder and cumulative damage to the brain. These studies also show a reduction of nerve cells in various areas of the brain. Research is beginning to find that lithium treatment is neurotrophic and neuro-protective, leading to increases in brain matter and nerve growth functions.

Neuropsychopharmacological research involving neuroimaging, MRI in particular, has also found initial evidence that lithium may counteract the reductions in gray-matter volume caused by bipolar disorder by providing a unique mechanism that increases hippocampal volume. It may be that despite lithium's toxicity—a primary reason for its stigma and lack of compliance—its restorative and protective effects will become its hallmark and its unique properties a reason for a new, more valued status.

And yet this research may make its way into commercial pharmaceutical laboratories, where already various much more expensive and less-tested atypical drugs have been produced for the market. All offer alternatives to lithium: Zyprexa, Seroquel, Lamictal, and, my favorite, Abilify. In the 2009 advertisement for Abilify, the message is that Abilify will manage symptoms so "you" can move ahead. Abilify will help you "move forward." Abilify is, of course, "clinically proven" to help control symptoms. And you are not alone, because hundreds of thousands of adult patients have been prescribed Abilify. This is the drug "for the road ahead." On the back page of the ad, the reader is told that Abilify may be taken alone—or with lithium. However, lithium, as a natural element, a single compound labeled generic, remains itself unpatentable and cannot bring in the money that newer mood stabilizers do. There is therefore no marketing strategy to deliver a new lithium with a new vocabulary. Who wouldn't want to be Abilified? Abled again? And who wouldn't want to be calmed by Seroquel or energized by Zyprexa? So much better, so many must think, than to be "flattened" or toxified by lithium. How much would we pay to be medicated by an all-purpose drug with no singular link to mania, no toxicity, no mystery?

The pharmacology and neuropharmacology of lithium treatment stretches mania almost to fragmentation. The language used by neurological studies is medicalized by talk of brain damage and nerve degeneration as much as neuroprotective properties—hardly the narrative we want to live with. We need a way to speak about lithium and mania that will allow us to live with drugs outside the languages of both madness and medicalization. We need a metaphor that will guide us out of the dystopian acceptance of a dangerous pharmaceutical complex and away from the utopian vision for a pharmaceutical cure. And we will need a vocabulary that will hold in the age of neuropsychopharmacology.

Neuro Futures: Posthuman or Multiple Beings?

As for a neuro future full of posthumans, there are those who would point out that we are already posthuman. Rather than imagine some natural essential humanness about us that will guarantee our freedom to control who we are as *ourselves*, we might acknowledge that what is already most characteristic of humanity in the neuro future is a merger of technology and the human. The vision is not one of a loss of the human but of "multiple ways of being embodied."[30] Advocates of alternative visions argue that human bodies have become hybrids. Rather than attempt to stay with the myth of "the human," it may be time to recognize and understand what it means to tell a different story about mingling or multiplying. We might even move beyond hybridity to multiplicity and begin to raise new questions. How will we live as multiples? What kind of multiple beings will we become? How will we perform multiply?

If mania is understood in light of multiplicity, it is not at all surprising that it would be more than one. And if the representation of the maniac comes to be represented as a multiple being, it would not be strange for that figure to be simultaneously mad and mentally ill. I've argued throughout the book that there is no "real" mania, not one defined in textbooks, not one that can be judged by morals, not something that can be identified in a gene or a molecule or neurotransmitter, and not even one that can be identified in the experiences of those diagnosed. This does not mean that mania isn't real. Mania coexists with madness even when it is medicalized as mental illness. So mania is neither merely madness nor fully medical, but both/and.

All construals of potential neuro futures note that things will definitely not be the same. There are successful meditations allowing for agnostic analysis of potential futures, avoiding any prediction of a radical shift to posthumanism or transhumanism. Nikolas Rose notes that the brain is the space of the gaze—but a different gaze from that of the nineteenth and the first half of the twentieth centuries. This is the space of visualization of cerebral tissue. This is the gaze, according to Rose, of biopower: change will come in small, and not always bad, mutations between life and politics. We are already, after all, in the space of visualization and are all "neurochemical selves."[31] In the space of visualization and neurochemical selves that Rose identifies, not only have entities such as receptor sites, synapses, and ion channels already come into being, but they have come into imaging color, so that bipolar brains are animated in yellow, green, and blue to show the cycles of illness during phases of bipolar disorder. As imaging technologies continue to assemble, the brain will only become more neurochemical, multilayered with fluids, radiation, and so on.

I began this book by suggesting that what we will all live with depends in part on how we decide to speak. Certainly, the language of neuropsychiatry can be reductive—dangerously so. Perhaps we will learn to emphasize both the challenges of coming to an understanding of the multifaceted activities in the brain, and the importance of delimiting studies to include other kinds of connections to technology, culture, and society. We need alternative rhetorics that leave us with more productive narratives. For example, in working with global accounts of psychiatry, diagnosis of bipolar disorder, and global pharmaceuticals, Andrew Lakoff ends with these questions: "Could knowledge of the psyche be assimilated into the new molecular sciences? What would such an effort mean for the politics of mental health? And what new position would the process imply for the subject of psychic distress?"[32] I too have no doubt that the neuro future leaves a great deal to be articulated and will be performed in ways we have yet to discover.

The coordination for centuries and among so many practices of mania as both madness and mental illness is a remarkable phenomenon. The story, however remarkable, ought to remind us that no single master narrative fits every case. If it appears as though I am arguing *for* one particular rhetoric of mania, it may be because I am, of course, arguing for multiple rhetorics—multiple histories and multiple futures. Without that acknowledgement, it would be impossible to move to the next step by identifying which words work, what combination of sentences ought to be articulated, and how we will choose to come into being as multiple beings.

EPILOGUE

A Mad, Mad World

Medical historians have noted that it was customary to describe the nineteenth century as "the nervous century."[1] The clinical term for "the nerves" was "neurasthenia," a condition marked by fatigue, headaches, indigestion, listlessness, and impoverished sexual activity. George Beard, member of the College of Physicians, began lecturing on the impoverished nervous system in the United States in 1868, describing various symptoms of neurasthenia. S. Weir Mitchell, who wrote extensively on the subject of public hygiene, in 1899 singled out the connection of neurasthenia to "mental hygiene," intending to identify a cause.

> That in one or another way the cruel competition for the dollar, the new and exacting habits of business, the racing speed which the telegraph and railway have introduced into commercial life, the value which great fortunes have come to possess as means toward social advancement, and the overeducation and overstraining of our young people have brought about some great and growing evils, is what is now beginning to be distinctly felt. I should like therefore at the risk of being tedious, to re-examine this question—to see if it be true that the nervous system of certain classes of Americans is being sorely overtaxed—and to ascertain how much our habits, our modes of work, and haply, climatic peculiarities, may have to do with the state of things.[2]

The state of "neurasthenia" was now linked to the modernization of American life, the excessive excitement of civilization.

Throughout the twentieth century, however, nerves were heightened by anxiety attacks to such a degree that W. H. Auden named the modern era the "Age of Anxiety." The elevation of neurasthenia to modern anxiety disorder as a distinctive clinical condition can be dated to 1895.[3] After the First World War and for most of the twentieth century, both veterans and civilians experienced

anxious expectation or neurotic anticipation accompanied by physical symptoms like cardiological and respiratory disturbance, tremors, chills, sweats, and
night terrors.

By the mid–twentieth century, what had first been considered "war neurosis"
had come to be considered a free-floating anxiety illness that affected a large portion of Americans and appeared to be a normal part of life. Again, this anxiety
has been attributed to contemporary standards of material consumption and
social status, technical change and economic growth, medical science and major
epidemic diseases, pathologic agents and radioactive gas, personal attractiveness
and physical defects, according to Michael Clark, who asks whether today's
ubiquitous condition of extreme anxiety means that we have moved "from the
'Age of Anxiety' to an Era of Panic."[4]

While anxiety may be considered a normal experience, its more extreme
manifestation—panic—is considered catastrophic; Clark describes it as "the
sudden and complete breakdown and collapse of individuals or whole societies
in the face of extraordinary or overwhelming pressures."[5] The history of panic is
sparse. In 1980, the term "panic disorder" was first used to describe recurrent
episodes of psychic terror. Jackie Orr, in *Panic Diaries: A Genealogy of Panic
Disorder*, situates panic in "the entangled fields of social science and psychiatry,
the U. S. Government and the military, the mass media and the transnational
drug industry."[6] Her work in the book is to relocate panic as a technosocial construction. Orr also takes note that where panic was once situated in historically
specific and collective behavior, the disorder is now understood as "generalized"—episodes occur without any discernable stimulus from social forces.

The anxious and frantic voice making itself heard in *Panic Diaries* bears
witness to panic as a "temporal disorder."[7] Has the "era of panic" notched up yet
again so that we are in the middle of another "temporal disorder"—a manic
phase? Two popular books, both published in 2005—*American Mania*, by
Peter C. Whybrow, and *The Hypomanic Edge*, by John D. Gartner—argue that
the United States historically and presently exhibits hypo/mania. Whybrow
writes as a practicing psychiatrist and director of the Neuropsychiatric Institute
at UCLA. His view of the nation in the twenty-first century is dark; he describes
the country's increased frenzy as "a dysfunctional state of mind that begins with
a joyous sense of excitement and high productivity but escalates into reckless
pursuit, irritability, and confusion." According to Whybrow, "unwittingly, in
our relentless pursuit of happiness we have overshot the target and spawned
a manic society with an insatiable appetite for more."[8] He identifies the causes
as linked to a changing economy, corporate greed, turbocharged lifestyles, and
commercial illusion. Whybrow suggests that his analogy to mania will generate
analysis that will help the United States escape from its otherwise inevitable,
uncontrollable fate.

However, Gartner, a professor of psychiatry at Johns Hopkins University,
reminds us that "mania" is more than a figure of speech. He suggests that

successful entrepreneurs are not manic and thus "not crazy." These people are, however, in his clinical estimation, "hypomanic." Gartner defines mania as a severe illness resulting in hospitalization or another external control for safety's sake, marked by bizarre, psychotic, dangerous, frightening, and disruptive behavior.[9] He defines hypomania, however, as a state on the border between abnormal and normal marked by energy, drive, optimism, and "Yankee ingenuity." Gartner proposes that hypomania could just as easily be "understood as expressions of *American temperament*."[10] Whether mania is a dangerous state of mind affecting collective social behavior, or a potentially less dangerous liminal state between normal and abnormal that serves the interest of Americans seeking success, the representation of mania in these two popular books by authors with psychiatric credibility is one of a frenzied, excited mind, still marked by excess. Emily Martin nicely describes the current affinity in U.S. culture for manic behavior, from popular television programs and music to newspaper articles and leadership books. As she documents public media's use of the word "mania," she notes, it has a nearly "positive gloss."[11]

The World Health Organization has identified bipolar disorder as the sixth leading cause of disability among all disorders for people between fifteen and forty-four. And yet bipolar disorder is the most undertreated psychiatric condition. Estimates suggest that only one-third of those suffering from bipolar disorder are ever properly diagnosed, and even fewer are treated. Prognosis is poor in comparison to most other psychiatric conditions. A third of individuals with bipolar disorder will attempt suicide sometime during their lives. Almost 50 percent of those diagnosed with bipolar disorder relapse within a year after recovery from a major episode. Even with appropriate, effective medication and management, three-quarters of those diagnosed with bipolar disorder will likely relapse at least once over a five-year period. Most individuals who successfully manage this condition will nevertheless experience symptoms between major depressive and manic episodes. It is estimated that those living with the condition lose fourteen functional, productive years and a full nine years of life. Bipolar disorder in children is becoming a more frequent and more controversial diagnosis. It is likely that the diagnostic criteria for bipolar disorder in both adults and children will be central to the next revision of the *Diagnostic Statistical Manual* (version V, expected to be available in 2012).[12]

As mania transitions fully into the twenty-first century and is altered again by a new textbook definition in the 2012 *DSM-V*, how will mania as the American temperament be expressed in the inclusion or exclusion of a diagnosis of childhood bipolar disorder? Until very recently, children were rarely diagnosed with bipolar disorder. Now, according to the National Alliance for Mental Illness, "although once thought rare, caseloads of patients examined for federally funded studies have shown that approximately 7 percent of children seen at psychiatric facilities fit the research standards for bipolar disorder."[13] Bipolar disorder has been investigated in children as young as six years old.

The concern regarding a diagnosis of bipolar disorder in children was inflamed after a two-year-old reportedly died from overmedication with drugs prescribed for bipolar disorder. *Frontline*'s coverage of childhood bipolar disorder, titled "The Medicated Child," only fueled public dismay regarding this diagnosis and its treatment by the psychiatric community.[14] Unfortunately, as more attention is focused on misdiagnosis or overmedication for bipolar disorder in children, less attention is paid to children who do exhibit symptoms of mania and depression. The film *Boy Interrupted* documents the life of a boy with bipolar disorder from childhood to adolescence and captures his day-to-day struggle at home, with friends, and at school. After a long period on and then off lithium, he commits suicide, jumping from his bedroom window.[15] Some findings indicate that children with bipolar disorder have a high rate of suicidal behavior and more severe features of bipolar illness than do adults.

The psychiatric community does not disagree that children and adolescents exhibit symptoms that might appear to constitute bipolar disorder, including severely unstable moods and extended periods of irritability. However, there is some disagreement as to whether large numbers of youth exhibit the classic symptoms of bipolar disorder, especially episodes of mania, and thus whether they ought to be diagnosed with this disorder. The questions seem to be: Is bipolar disorder one thing, and mania its defining manifestation? Or does bipolar disorder affect different populations, including children, differently, and might mania also, then, be a different thing for children?

Some professionals believe that children with chronic severe irritability, emotional instability, and agitated outbursts to the extent that they are impaired should be diagnosed with bipolar disorder and treated accordingly. Others argue that using watered-down criteria, and criteria that children may exhibit normally in the course of their development, will result in overdiagnosis and overtreatment with unfortunate side effects and long-term brain function implications. The American Psychiatric Association (APA) is proposing a revision to the *DSM-V* that would navigate this controversy. The APA Child and Adolescent Disorders Work Group has suggested a new category for children who do not fit the criteria for mania—temper dysregulation disorder with dysphoria—to better diagnose children who have some symptoms of bipolar disorder but do not have clear manic episodes.[16] This working group does not intend to replace childhood bipolar disorder and is not arguing that children cannot exhibit the full range of symptoms of bipolar disorder. However, it does argue that children have been misdiagnosed and overdiagnosed with bipolar disorder because of the lack of a more accurate alternative.

According to the report, temper dysregulation disorder with dysphoria is characterized by "severe recurrent temper outbursts in response to common stressors" that manifest as "verbal rages" with "physical aggression" that are "grossly out of proportion." The "mood between temper outbursts is persistently negative (irritable, angry, and/or sad)." Explicit criteria state that there must be an absence of abnormally elevated or expansive mood, defined as "grandiosity or inflated self esteem, decreased need for sleep, pressured speech, flight of ideas, distractibility, increase in goal directed activity, or excessive involvement in activities with a high potential for painful consequences." The APA is being careful to distinguish this disorder from normal "temper tantrums" and bad moods. When the draft of the new *DSM* was released to the public in a press release on February 10, 2010, Dr. David Shaffer of the work group cautioned that temper dysregulation disorder with dysphoria is very different in frequency and impact from what parents see in normal development: "These are children whose outbursts may injure siblings, parents and schoolteachers," he said. "They may cause extensive damage to property, and the impact of their symptoms on family life is quite profound. It is not uncommon for such children to require psychiatric hospitalization." The Child and Adolescent Disorders Work Group continues to work on possible modifications to pediatric bipolar disorder, and new criteria for mania may emerge.[17]

The Child and Adolescent Bipolar Foundation, however, has rightly objected to the name of the proposed diagnosis, arguing that "temper dysregulation disorder" conjures the wrong image for children. The foundation focuses on the word "temper" and expresses concern that the child will be seen as "brattish." The distinction from the bipolar diagnosis, on the other hand, "allows for the possibility that these children will not be burdened by a lifelong illness."[18] While the foundation is smart to target the name of the disorder, the emphasis on severing the relationship to bipolar disorder could be taken as a conflict in working against the stigma of mental illness. My own reading of this proposed revision notes the defined criteria as gross "rages" with "physical aggression" with "persistently negative (irritable, angry, and/or sad)" mood. I also note Shaffer's description of violent behavior that is apt to injure others and damage property. The old raging fury of madness is merely surrounded by familiar sentences, making up yet another kind of madness. Temper dysregulation disorder with dysphoria is distinguished from bipolar disorder only in its characterization as purely dysphoric or as lacking euphoria. Its definition does little to convince that one or the other will be more or less coordinated with mania's making in its afterlife.

The remnants of classical madness entangled in clinical mania and mental illness remain discomforting for me as I read diagnostic descriptions that highlight extreme irritation, excessive activity, aggression, and rage. For the APA and mental health organizations to claim that such depictions of madness have vanished or have been replaced by more reasonable clinical encounters of illness is to make it even more difficult for me to evaluate my symptoms (or lack thereof) or to consider strategies for negotiating options for action.

Where will the thousands and thousands of parents of suffering children or the millions of suffering adults turn if they do not recognize the violent rage or delusional flights of fancy in these categories? Given the persistence of classical madness and its infusion in mental illness, there is no easy plan by which to interrupt the discursive descriptions of mania, whether in its inclusion or by exclusion. How manic identities will be forged and contested in what will likely be permanent chaos depends on where the tensions traced out in this book take us next. The new edition of the *DSM* does not, and likely cannot, be a space in which to undertake the kind of interruption necessary.

There are different, multiple ways of talking with mania and about mania, and it is all very messy. The profound rhetorical changes that will be needed to intervene in social and biological worlds will not happen without an understanding of the patterns described in this book. Even so, determining whether any interruption is a good one will prove difficult, and will not be immediately obvious. The best we can do is what we've done here: treat mania as an object that is elusive, always *in potentia* and yet always hard to make go away. We can only document how mania is manipulated and how it multiplies to remain so tenacious an object that, even when altered, it sustains its history in its emergence. After all that, can we enact mania in a better way—a good way?

NOTES

INTRODUCTION

1. Andrew Skull, *Social Order/Social Disorder: Anglo-American Psychiatry in Historical Perspective* (Berkeley: University of California Press, 1989), 58.

2. G. E. Berrios, "Classic Text No. 57: Of Mania: (from Bucknill and Tuke, 1858)," *History of Psychiatry* 15.1 (2004): 109; G. E. Berrios, "Mood Disorders," in *A History of Clinical Psychiatry: The Origin and History of Psychiatric Disorders*, ed. German Berrios and Roy Porter (New Brunswick, N.J.: Athlone Press, 1995), 384–408.

3. David Loring, ed., *INS Dictionary of Neuropsychiatry* (New York: Oxford University Press, 1999), 102.

4. Sotiris Kotsopoulos, "Aretaeus the Cappadocian on Mental Illness," *Comprehensive Psychiatry* 27.2 (1986): 176.

Various clinicians and historians have attributed more or less significance to the origin of the concept in Aretaeus and its subsequent evolution to its status as a modern medical term. Berrios has written frequently on this subject. See, e.g., Berrios, "Mood Disorders: Clinical Section," in *A History of Clinical Psychiatry: The Origin and History of Psychiatric Disorders*, ed. German Berrios and Roy Porter (New Brunswick, N.J.: Athlone Press, 1995), 384. See also: Kotsopoulos, "Aretaeus the Cappadocian on Mental Illness," 171–179.

5. American Psychiatric Association, *Diagnostic and Statistical Manual of Mental Disorders: DSM-IV-TR* (Washington, D.C.: American Psychiatric Association, 2000): 357–358.

6. See discussion in Marcel Gauchet and Gladys Swain, *Madness and Democracy: The Modern Psychiatric Universe*, trans. Catherine Porter (Princeton: Princeton University Press, 1999), 232.

7. Ibid.

8. Michel Foucault, *History of Madness*, ed. Jean Khalfa, trans. Jonathan Murphy and Jean Khalfa (London: Routledge, 2006), 503.

9. Ibid., 504.

10. Jean Baudrillard, Sylvère Lotringer, and Nicole Dufresne, *Forget Foucault*, rev. ed. (1970; repr., Los Angeles: Semiotext, 2007), 30.

11. Ian Hacking, *Historical Ontology* (Cambridge, Mass.: Harvard University Press, 2002), 17.

12. Annemarie Mol, *The Body Multiple: Ontology in Medical Practice* (Durham, N.C.: Duke University Press, 2002).

13. See, e.g., Edward Hare, "The Two Manias: A Study of the Evolution of the Modern Concept of Mania," *British Journal of Psychiatry* 138 (1981): 89–99; O. Diethelm, "Mania: A Clinical Study of Dissertations before 1750," *Confinia Psychiatrica* 13.9 (1970): 26–49; Berrios, "Classic Text," 105–124.

14. David Healy, *Mania: A Short History of Bipolar Disorder* (Baltimore: Johns Hopkins University Press, 2008).

15. Peter Conrad and Joseph W. Schneider, *Deviance and Medicalization: From Badness to Sickness*, 3d ed. (Philadelphia: Temple University Press, 1981), 7.

16. John Law and Annemarie Mol, eds., *Complexities: Social Studies of Knowledge Practices* (Durham, N.C.: Duke University Press, 2002).

17. Emily Martin, *Bipolar Expeditions: Mania and Depression in American Culture* (Princeton, N.J.: Princeton University Press, 2007).

18. Jackie Orr, *Panic Diaries: A Genealogy of Panic Disorder* (Durham, N.C.: Duke University Press, 2006); Jonathan Metzel, *Prozac on the Couch: Prescribing Gender in the Era of Wonder Drugs* (Durham, N.C.: Duke University Press, 2003); Janet Wirth-Cauchon, *Women and Borderline Personality Disorder: Symptoms and Stories* (New Brunswick, N.J.: Rutgers University Press, 2001).

19. Len Bowers, *The Social Nature of Mental Illness* (New York: Routledge, 1998), 159–160.

20. Lorraine Daston, ed., *Biographies of Scientific Objects* (Chicago: University of Chicago Press, 2000); John Law, *After Method: Mess in Social Science Research* (London: Routledge, 2004); John Law and Vicky Singleton. "Performing Technology's Stories: On Social Constructivism, Performance, and Performativity," *Technology and Culture* 41.4 (2000): 765–775; Charis Thompson, *Making Parents: The Ontological Choreography of Reproductive Technologies* (Cambridge, Mass.: MIT Press, 2005); Isabelle Baszanger, *Inventing Pain Medicine: From the Laboratory to the Clinic* (New Brunswick, N.J: Rutgers University Press, 1998).

21. Andy Clark, *Natural-born Cyborgs: Minds, Technologies, and the Future of Human Intelligence* (Oxford: Oxford University Press, 2003), 180.

CHAPTER 1 — MANIA MULTIPLIES WITH FURY

1. Edward Shorter, *A History of Psychiatry: From the Era of the Asylum to the Age of Prozac* (New York: John Wiley and Sons, 1997), 13.

2. Etienne Esquirol, *Mental Maladies: A Treatise on Insanity* (Philadelphia: Lee and Blanchard, 1845), 395.

3. Mania is understood throughout this book as socially manipulated, linguistically captured, and materially assembled. When referring to mania being constructed, I mean to say that it is performed in cultural, discursive, and embodied ways.

4. Emil Kraepelin, *Manic Depressive Insanity and Paranoia* (Edinburgh: Livingstone, 1921), and *Compendium der Psychiatrie* (Leipzig: A. Abel, 1883).

5. For justification of a method of mapping that accounts for complexities without handling a comprehensive endeavor, see John Law and Annemarie Mol, *Complexities: Social Studies of Knowledge Practices* (Durham, N.C.: Duke University Press, 2002).

6. Charles E. Goshen, ed., *Documentary History of Psychiatry* (New York: Philosophical Library, 1967), 6.

7. Aretaeus, *Aretaeus: The Extant Works*, ed. and trans. Adams F. London, Sydenham Society (Boston: Longwood Press, 1978), 303, qtd. in Sotiris Kotsopoulos, "Aretaeus the Cappadocian on Mental Illness," *Comprehensive Psychiatry* 27.2 (1986): 176.

8. Caelius Aurelianus, "Madness or Insanity (Greek: Mania)," in *Documentary History of Psychiatry*, ed. Charles E. Goshen (New York: Philosophical Library, 1967), 18–31.

9. G. E. Berrios, "Mood Disorders," in *A History of Clinical Psychiatry: The Origin and History of Psychiatric Disorders*, ed. German Berrios and Roy Porter (London: Athlone Press, 1995), 388.

10. J.F.C. Hecker, *The Dancing Mania of the Middle Ages* (New York: B. Franklin, 1970), 540.

11. Ibid., 3.

12. Paracelsus, "Diseases That Deprive Man of His Reason," in *Documentary History of Psychiatry*, ed. Charles E. Goshen (New York: Philosophical Library, 1967), 46.

13. Felix Platter, "Histories and Observations upon Most Diseases," trans. Cole and Culper (London: 1662), qtd. in O. Diethelm, "Mania: A Clinical Study of Dissertations before 1750," *Confinia Psychiatria* 13 (1970): 27–28.

14. Thomas Willis, *Dr. Willis's Practice of Physik: Being the Whole Works of That Renowned and Famous Physician* (London: C. Harper and J. Leight, 1648), 201.

15. Hermann Boerhaave, "Of the Maniacal or Roving Madness," in *Documentary History of Psychiatry*, ed. Charles E. Goshen (New York: Philosophical Library, 1967), 230.

16. William Cullen, *First Lines of the Practice of Physic* (Edinburgh: C. Elliot, 1784), 4:145–146.

17. William Pargeter, *Observations on Maniacal Disorders* (Reading, 1792), ed. Stanley W. Jackson (London: Routledge, 1988).

18. Philippe Pinel, *A Treatise on Insanity: In Which Are Contained the Principles of a New and More Practical Nosology of Maniacal Disorders Than Has Yet Been Offered to the Public*, trans. D. D. Davis (The Strand, London: W. Todd for Cadell and Davies, 1806), 150.

19. Esquirol, *Mental Maladies*, 377–378.

20. Ibid., 378, 385, 378.

21. Ibid., 387.

22. M. J. Sedler, "Falret's Discovery: The Origin of the Concept of Bipolar Affective Disorder," trans. Mark Sedler and Eric C. Dessain, *American Journal of Psychiatry* 140.9 (September 1983): 1130. The text is translated from Jean Pierre Falret, "Memoire sur la folie circulaire" (Memoir on circular insanity), 1854.

23. John Charles Bucknill and Daniel H. Tuke, *A Manual of Psychological Medicine*, 3d ed. (Philadelphia: Lindsay and Blakiston, 1874), 296, 297.

24. Ibid., 307.

25. First published in 1883, the Commendium was edited consistently through its definitive sixth edition in 1899.

26. Emil Kraepelin and A. R. Diefendorf, *Clinical Psychiatry: A Text-Book for Students and Physicians*, in *Lifetime Editions of Kraepelin in English*, vol. 2 (Bristol: Thoemmes Press, 2002). Abstracted and adapted from the seventh German edition of Kraepelin's "Lehrbuch der Psychiatrie."

27. Emil Kraepelin, *Manic Depressive Insanity and Paranoia* (Edinburgh: Livingstone, 1921), 6, 23. Succeeding references to this work are cited by page number in the text.

28. Great controversies within clinical and research psychiatry and among certain public groups affected by the revisions, particularly revisions regarding sexual deviance, are covered in several texts. See Stuart A. Kirk and Herb Kutchins, *The Selling of the DSM: The Rhetoric of Science in Psychiatry* (Hawthorne, N.Y.: Aldine de Gruyter, 1992), for a nice introduction to the arguments.

29. American Psychiatric Association, *Diagnostic and Statistical Manual of Mental Disorders: DSM-IV-TR* (Washington, D.C.: American Psychiatric Association, 2000), 357.

30. Ibid., 357–358.

31. For the term "psy-sciences," see Andrew Lakoff, *Pharmaceutical Reason: Knowledge and Value in Global Psychiatry* (New York: Cambridge University Press, 2005), 3.

32. Sigmund Freud, "Mourning and Melancholia," in *Standard Edition of the Complete Psychological Works of Sigmund Freud*, vol. 14, ed. and trans. James Strachey (London: Hogarth Press, 1957), 254.

33. Roy Porter, "Mood Disorders," in *History of Clinical Psychiatry: The Origin and History of Psychiatric Diseases*, ed. G. E. Berrios and Roy Porter (Linton: Athlone, 1995), 419. Porter makes a distinction between various neuroses and the maniac as psychotic.

34. Edward Shorter, *A History of Psychiatry: From the Asylum to the Age of Prozac* (New York: John Wiley and Sons, 1997).

35. Jonathan Michel Metzel, *Prozac on the Couch: Prescribing Gender in the Era of Wonder Drugs* (Durham, N.C.: Duke University Press, 2003).

36. Alfred M. Freedman, Harold I. Kaplan, and Benjamin J. Sadock, *Comprehensive Textbook of Psychiatry, II* (Baltimore: Williams and Wilkins, 1975), 1018A.

37. Ibid., 1018A.

38. Ibid.

39. G. L. Klerman, "The Spectrum of Mania," *Comprehensive Psychiatry* 22 (1981): 11–20; D. L. Dunner, "Clinical Consequences of Under-Recognized Bipolar Spectrum Disorder," *Bipolar Disorder* 5 (2003): 456–463; Hagop S. Akiskal, "The Prevalent Clinical Spectrum of Bipolar Disorders: Beyond DSM-IV," *Journal of Clinical Psychopharmacology* 62 (1996): 4S–14S.

40. Dunner, "Clinical Consequences," 458.

41. Guy Goodwin, "Hypomania: What's in a Name?" *British Journal of Psychiatry* 181 (2002): 94–95.

42. Ronald R. Fieve, *Bipolar II: Enhance Your Highs, Boost Your Creativity, and Escape the Cycles of Recurrent Depression* (New York: Rodale, 2006), book jacket.

43. Lana R. Castle, *Finding Your Bipolar Muse: How to Master Depressive Droughts and Manic Floods and Access Your Creative Power* (New York: Marlowe, 2006).

44. Nancy C. Andreasen, *Brave New Brain: Conquering Mental Illness in the Era of the Genome* (Oxford: Oxford University Press, 2001); Kay R. Jamison, *An Unquiet Mind* (New York: Knopf, 1995).

45. Akiskal, "Prevalent Clinical Spectrum"; Hagop Akiskal, Marc L. Bourgeois, Jules Angst, Robert Post, Hans-Jürgen Möller, and Robert Hirschfeld, "Re-Evaluating the Prevalence of and Diagnostic Composition within the Broad Clinical Spectrum of Bipolar Disorders," *Journal of Affective Disorders* 59 (2000): S5–S30.

46. Benjamin J, Sadock and Virginia A. Sadock, *Comprehensive Textbook of Psychiatry* (Philadelphia: Lippincott Williams and Wilkins, 2000), 1348.

47. Michael Gelder, Nancy Andreasen, Juan Lopez-Ibor, and John Geddes, eds., *New Oxford Textbook of Psychiatry*, 2d ed. (Oxford: Oxford University Press, 2009).

CHAPTER 2 — THE MANIAC AND THE ICONOGRAPHY OF REFORM

1. Philippe Pinel, *Memoir on Madness*, 1794, qtd in. Debra B. Weiner, "Philippe Pinel's 'Memoir on Madness' of December 11, 1794: A Fundamental Text of Modern Psychiatry," *American Journal of Psychiatry* 149:6 (1992): 731.

2. Samuel Tuke, *Description of the Retreat, an Institution near York, for Insane Persons of the Society of Friends* (Philadelphia: Isaac Pierce, 1813), 94.

3. The canon of texts, in chronological order: Albert Deutsch, *The Mentally Ill in America: A History of Their Care and Treatment from Colonial Times* (1949); Thomas

Szasz, *The Myth of Mental Illness: Foundations of a Theory of Personal Conduct* (1961); Erving Goffman, *Asylums: Essays on the Social Situation of Mental Patients and Other Inmates* (1961); David J. Rothman, *The Discovery of the Asylum: Social Order and Disorder in the New Republic* (1971); Phyllis Chesler, *Women and Madness* (1972); Gerald Grob, *Mental Institutions in America: Social Policy to 1875* (1973); Andrew Scull, *The Museums of Madness: The Social Organization of Madness in Nineteenth-Century England* (1979).

4. Michel Foucault, *History of Madness*, ed. Jean Khalfa, trans. Jonathan Murphy and Jean Khalfa (New York: Routledge), 508, 487.

5. What Foucault called an "archeology" or genealogical history is a story about how madness as mental illness became an object of scientific study of the psyche—and in particular how individual minds and bodies then became the locus of cultural pathologies. Across Foucault's work on madness, our general malaise has been turned into a symptom of potentially dangerous repressed desire and our sexuality has been made available to inspection and correction by the power located in the practices of psychoanalysis.

6. Daniel Walker Howe, *What Hath God Wrought: The Transformation of America, 1815–1848* (New York: Oxford University Press, 2007), 55.

7. "Patients, Admissions, etc. 1752–1786," archives of the Pennsylvania Hospital, Philadelphia.

8. Ibid.

9. Ohio Lunatic Asylum, *Annual Report of the Directors of the Ohio Lunatic Asylum* (Columbus: Samuel Medary, printer to the state, 1839), 17.

10. For a thorough discussion of Thomas Kirkbride's ideals for asylum construction, see Nancy Tomes, *The Art of Asylum-Keeping: Thomas Story Kirkbride and the Origins of American Psychiatry* (Philadelphia: University of Pennsylvania Press, 1994).

11. For a thorough discussion of nineteenth-century asylum architecture, see Carla Yanni, *The Architecture of Madness: Insane Asylums in the United States* (Minneapolis: University of Minnesota Press, 2007).

12. David D. Hall, *Cultures of Print: Essays in the History of the Book* (Amherst: University of Massachusetts Press, 1996).

13. Tuke, *Description of the Retreat*, 94. Succeeding references to this work are cited by page number in the text.

14. *Appeal to the People of Pennsylvania on the Subject of an Asylum for the Insane Poor* (Philadelphia: Printed for the Committee, 1838), 19.

15. Tennessee Lunatic Asylum, *First Report of the Physician of the Tennessee Lunatic Asylum: To the Legislature of Tennessee, for 1840 and 1841* (Nashville: W. F. Bang, 1841), 10; Lunatic Asylum of South Carolina, *Report of the Committee of Regents, Report of the Physician, Report of the Superintendent, Laws of the Institution, etc.* (Columbia: Morgan Isaac, 1842), 5.

16. Boston Lunatic Hospital, *Report of the Superintendent of the Boston Lunatic Hospital and Physician of the Public Institution at South Boston* (Boston: John H. Eastburn, 1840), 13.

17. Contributors to the Asylum for the Relief of Persons Deprived of the Use of Their Reason, *Annual Report on the State of the Asylum for the Relief of Persons Deprived of the Use of Their Reason* (Philadelphia: Philadelphia Asylum, 1835).

18. Pennsylvania Hospital for the Insane, *Report of the Pennsylvania Hospital for the Insane* (Philadelphia: James C. Haswell, 1842), 22.

19. Ibid., 6, 40.

20. Pennsylvania Hospital for the Insane, *Annual Report of the Pennsylvania Hospital for the Insane* (Philadelphia: T. K. and P. G. Collins, printers, 1856), 7.

21. Mario Biagoli and Peter Galison, *Scientific Authorship: Credit and Intellectual Property in Science* (New York: Routledge, 2003).

22. Contributors to the Asylum for the Relief of Persons Derived of the Use of Their Reason, *Annual Report on the State of the Asylum for the Relief of Persons Derived of the Use of Their Reason* (Philadelphia: Philadelphia Asylum, 1848), 7

23. Ohio Lunatic Asylum, *Third Annual Report of the Directors of the Ohio Lunatic Asylum* (Columbus: n.p., 1837), 7.

24. State Asylum for New Jersey Lunatics, *Report of the Commissioners Appointed by the Governor of New Jersey to Ascertain the Number of Lunatics and Idiots in the State* (Newark: M. S. Harrison, 1840), 12, 23.

25. Joint Committee of Council and Assembly, Trenton, *Report Relative to an Asylum for Lunatics, by the Joint Committee of Council and Assembly* (Trenton, N.J.: Sherman and Harron, 1881), 3–4.

26. *Annual Report of the Trustees of the State Lunatic Hospital at Worcester* (Boston: Dutton and Wentworth, 1835), 20.

27. Lunatic Asylum of South Carolina, *Lunatic Asylum of South Carolina: Report of the Committee of Regents, Report of the Physician, Report of the Superintendent, Laws of the Institution, etc.* (Columbia: Morgan Isaac, 1842), 15.

28. Vermont State Asylum, *Twenty-Fifth Annual Report of the Officers of the Vermont Asylum for the Insane* (Brattleboro: George E. Selleck, printer, 1861), 9.

29. Vermont State Asylum, *Twenty-Seventh Annual Report of the Officers of the Vermont Asylum for the Insane* (Brattleboro: D. W. Selleck, printer, 1863); Iowa Hospital for the Insane (Mount Pleasant, Iowa), *Report of the Officers of the Iowa Hospital for the Insane to the Governor of the State of Iowa: For the Fiscal Years 1866–67* (Des Moines: F. W. Palmer, state printer, 1868), 16.

30. *Report of the Proceedings for Establishing a Board of Commissioners in Lunacy for the State of New York* (New York: A. G. Sherwood, 1880), 44, 12.

31. Western Lunatic Asylum, *Sixteenth Annual Report of the President and Directors of the Western Lunatic Asylum, to the Legislature of Virginia: With the Report of the Superintendent and Physician, for 1842* (Staunton, Va.: Printed at the Spectator Office, 1843), 35.

32. New York State Lunatic Asylum, *Annual Report of the Managers of the New York State Lunatic Asylum* (Albany: n.p., 1844), 13.

33. Western Lunatic Asylum, *Sixteenth Annual Report*, 4, 7.

34. New Hampshire Asylum for the Insane/George Chandler, *Reports of the Board of Visitors, of the Trustees, and of the Superintendent of the New Hampshire Asylum for the Insane: June Session, 1843* (Concord, N.H.: Carroll and Baker, 1843), 19.

35. Lunatic Asylum of South Carolina, *Lunatic Asylum of South Carolina: Report*, 7.

36. Eastern Lunatic Asylum, *Report of the Eastern Lunatic Asylum: In the City of Williamsburg, Virginia, 1851* (1852) reports thirty free colored and eight slaves housed in the asylum. Only admissions and statistical information regarding height, weight, and pulse were offered (as for every patient). For additional primary documents on the treatment of race in the nineteenth century, see Edward Jarvis, "Insanity among the Colored Population of the Free States," *American Journal of the Medical Sciences* 7 (1844): 71–83; and A. H. Witmer, "Insanity in the Colored Race in the United States," *Alienist and Neurologist* 12 (1891).

37. Eastern Lunatic Asylum, *Report, 1851*, 17.

38. State Asylum for New Jersey Lunatics, *Report of the Commissioners*, 9.

39. Ibid., *Report of the Managers*, 73.

40. New York State Lunatic Asylum, *Thirteenth Annual Report of the Managers of the New York State Lunatic Asylum* (Albany: C. Van Benthuysen, printer to the Legislature, 1856), 22, 10.

41. Vermont State Asylum, *Twenty-Fourth Annual Report of the Officers of the Vermont Asylum for the Insane* (Brattleboro: George E. Selleck, printer, 1860), 12.

42. Pennsylvania Hospital for the Insane, *Annual Report of the Pennsylvania Hospital for the Insane* (Philadelphia: Collins, printer, 1860), 10.

43. Illinois State Hospital for the Insane, *Ninth Biennial Report of the Trustees, Superintendent and Treasurer of the Illinois State Hospital for the Insane at Jacksonville* (Springfield: Baker and Phillips, printers, 1864).

44. *Report of the Proceedings*, 23.

45. Ohio Lunatic Asylum, *Annual Report*, 1.

46. Western Lunatic Hospital, *Report of the Physician*, 10.

47. State Asylum for New Jersey Lunatics, *Report of the Commissioners*, 11.

48. New Hampshire Asylum for the Insane/George Chandler, *Reports*, 20.

49. Samuel Hare, *Statistical Report of One Hundred and Ninety Cases of Insanity, Admitted into the Retreat near Leeds: Provincial Medical Journal* (London: S. Taylor, printer, 1843), 12.

50. Eastern Lunatic Asylum, *Report, 1851*, 24.

51. Illinois State Hospital for the Insane, *Ninth Biennial Report*.

52. State of New York, *Extract from the Ninth Annual Report of the State Board of Charities of the State of New York, Relating to Hospitals for the Sick and Insane* (Albany: Weed, Parsons, printers, 1876), 4.

53. Pennsylvania Hospital, *Annual Report*, 1896, 8.

54. New York State Lunatic Asylum, *Thirty-First Annual Report of the Managers of the New York State Lunatic Asylum* (Albany: Weed, Parsons, printers, 1873), 44.

55. Pennsylvania Hospital, *Report of the Pennsylvania Hospital for the Insane for the Year 1883* (Philadelphia: n.p., 1884), 30.

56. Pennsylvania Hospital for the Insane, *Annual Report*, 1860, 39.

57. Pennsylvania Hospital, *Annual Report of the Department for the Insane of the Pennsylvania Hospital* (Philadelphia: Press of Lehman and Bolton, 1891), 17

58. Dorothea L. Dix, *Memorial to the Legislature of Massachusetts* (1843; Lyrasis Members and Sloan Foundation, 2009), 5, http://www.archive.org/details/memorialtolegis100dixd.

59. Charles Dickens, *American Notes for General Circulation* (New York: Penguin Classics, 1985), 104, 54.

60. Ibid., 84.

61. Edgar Allan Poe, "The System of Doctor Tarr and Professor Fether" (1845; Baltimore: Edgar Allan Poe Society of Baltimore, 2008), http://www.eapoe.org/works/tales/tarrb.htm. It ought not escape attention that Poe's own sanity was questioned by Dr. Henry Maudsley, who concluded that Poe "was utterly destitute of the faculty of reasonable insight." Henry Maudsley, "Edgar Allen Poe," *Journal of Insanity* 17.2 (October 1860): 196–197.

62. David S. Reynolds, *Beneath the American Renaissance: The Subversive Imagination in the Age of Emerson and Melville* (Cambridge, Mass.: Harvard University Press, 1988), 59. Also see Michael Denning, *Mechanic Accents: Dime Novels and Working-Class Culture in America* (New York: Verso, 1987); Paul Joseph Erickson, "Welcome to Sodom: The Cultural Work of City-Mysteries Fiction in Antebellum America" (PhD diss., University

of Texas at Austin, 2005); Shelley Streeby, *American Sensations: Class, Empire, and the Production of Popular Culture* (Berkeley: University of California Press, 2002).

63. A.J.H. Duganne, *The Knights of the Seal; or, The Mysteries of the Three Cities: A Romance of Men's Hearts and Habits* (Philadelphia: Colon and Adriance, 1845), 19.

64. Ibid., 55, 204.

65. Philippe Pinel, *A Treatise on Insanity: In Which Are Contained the Principles of a New and More Practical Nosology of Maniacal Disorders Than Has Yet Been Offered to the Public,* trans. D. D. Davis (The Strand, London: W. Todd for Cadell and Davies, 1806), 251.

66. Foucault recognized this interpretation in the philanthropy of Couthon at work at Bicêtre Hospital, speculating that "madness had thus emigrated to the side of its keepers; those who locked up the mad like animals were now possessed by the animal brutality of insanity." Foucault, *History of Madness,* 477.

67. Michel Foucault, *Psychiatric Power: Lectures at the College de France, 1973–1974,* ed. Jacques Lagrange, trans. Graham Burchell (New York: Picador, 2006).

68. "Money-Making Mania," *Journal of Insanity* (April 1849), 327, 328.

69. Benjamin Reiss, *Theaters of Madness: Insane Asylums and Nineteenth-Century American Culture* (Chicago: University of Chicago Press, 2008), 14, 17.

CHAPTER 3 — MIDWESTERN MANIA

1. Marc Berg and Annemarie Mol, *Differences in Medicine: Unraveling Practices, Techniques, and Bodies* (Durham, N.C: Duke University Press, 1998), 5.

2. George Winokur and Ming T. Tsuang, *The Natural History of Mania, Depression, and Schizophrenia* (Washington, D.C.: American Psychiatric Press, 1996), 2.

3. Ibid., 35.

4. Martin Alda, "In Memoriam: Professor George Winokur," *Journal of Psychiatry and Neuroscience* 22 (January 1997): 70.

5. Staffan Müller-Wille and Hans-Jörg Rheinberger, *Heredity Produced: At the Crossroads of Biology, Politics, and Culture, 1500–1870* (Cambridge, Mass: MIT Press, 2007), 18–19.

6. Phillip Thurtle, *The Emergence of Genetic Rationality: Space, Time, and Information in American Biological Science, 1870–1920* (Seattle: University of Washington Press, 2007), 6.

7. E. N. Smith, C. S. Bloss, J. A. Badner, T. Barrett, P. L. Belmonte, W. Berrettini, W. Byerley, W. Coryell, D. Craig, H. J. Edenberg, E. Eskin, et al. "Genome-wide Association Study of Bipolar Disorder in European American and African American Individuals," *Molecular Psychiatry* 14.8 (2009): 755–763.

8. D. L. M'Gugin, "Cases in Practice," *Iowa Medical Journal* (August/September 1855): 327; ibid., "Outraged Laws of Hygiene," *Iowa Medical Journal* (June/July 1855): 413.

9. Iowa Hospital for the Insane (Mount Pleasant, Iowa), *Report of the Officers of the Iowa Hospital for the Insane to the Governor of the State of Iowa: For the Fiscal Years 1866–67* (Des Moines: F.W. Palmer, state printer, 1868).

10. Hospital for the Insane at Independence, *First Biennial Report of the Hospital for the Insane at Independence* (Des Moines: Hospital for the Insane at Independence, 1874).

11. Gershom H. Hill, "Prognosis in Insanity," *Iowa Medical Journal* (October 1895): 381.

12. Iowa Board of Control of State Institutions, *Biennial Report of the Board of Control of State Institutions of Iowa* (Des Moines: State printer, June 1914), 302.

13. Ibid., *State of Iowa Bulletin of State Institutions* (Anamosa, Iowa: Reformatory Press, 1922).

14. Ibid., 129. Succeeding references to this bulletin are cited by page number in the text.

15. *Acts of the Thirty-Fourth General Assembly of Iowa*, July 4, 1911, Chapter 129. The law was repealed and substituted for by Chapter 187, *Acts of the Thirty-Fifth General Assembly*, April 19, 1913.

16. See Amy Vogel, "Regulating Degeneracy: Eugenic Sterilization in Iowa, 1911–1977," *Annals of Iowa* 54 (1995): 121–143. For discussions of eugenics in the *Journal of the Iowa State Medical Society*, see "Legalized Eugenic Sterilization," *JISMS* 25 (1935): 155; "Report of Special Committee on Eugenics," *JISMS* 11 (1921): 278; "Sterilization of the Unfit," *JISMS* 19 (1929): 127–128; Eleanor Hutchinson, "Possibilities for Race Betterment," *JISMS* 24 (1934): 577–580; Willard C. Brinegar et al., "Sterilization of Patients Discharged from Four Iowa State Hospitals in 1947," *JISMS* 40 (1950): 263–264.

17. Harry H. Laughlin, "Report of the Committee to Study and to Report on the Best Practical Means of Cutting Off the Defective Germ-Plasm in the American Population: The Scope of the Committee's Work" (College of Law Faculty Publications, Paper 10, 2009), 25, http://digitalarchive.gsu.edu/col_facpub/10.

18. Thurtle, *The Emergence of Genetic Rationality*.

19. Winokur and Tsuang, *Natural History*, 19. Succeeding references to this work are cited by page number in the text.

20. Winokur, *Mania and Depression*, 30, 14–15.

21. Ibid., 35.

22. Winokur engaged a wide network of research collaborators and was author or coauthor of nearly three hundred articles during his career, from 1965 to 1996.

23. In *Pharmaceutical Reason: Knowledge and Value in Global Psychiatry* (Cambridge: Cambridge University Press, 2005), Andrew Lakoff posits the question, Could there be a "gene-for" bipolar disorder, and would discourse, research, and pharmacological treatment stabilize the disorder into a durable entity?

24. Smith et al., "Genome-wide Association Study," 175. Succeeding references to this work are cited by page number in the text.

25. Nikolas Rose, *The Politics of Life Itself: Biomedicine, Power, and Subjectivity in the Twenty-First Century* (Princeton, N.J.: Princeton University Press, 2006).

26. Smith et al., "Genome-wide Association Study."

27. National Human Genome Research Institute, "Personalized Medicine: How the Human Genome Era Will Usher in a Health Care Revolution," http://www.genome.gov/13514107.

28. Sahotra Sarkar, "From Genes as Determinants to DNA as Resource," in *Genes in Development: Re-Reading the Molecular Paradigm*, ed. Eva M. Neumann-Held and Christoph Rehmann-Sutter (Durham, N.C.: Duke University Press, 2006), 86.

CHAPTER 4 — MANIC LIVES

1. Andy Behrman, *Electroboy: A Memoir of Mania* (New York: Random House, 2002), xix. Succeeding references to this work are cited by page number in the text.

2. Patty Duke and Gloria Hochman, *A Brilliant Madness: Living with Manic-Depressive Illness* (New York: Bantam Books, 1992); Jane Pauley, *Skywriting: A Life out of the Blue* (New York: Random House, 2004).

3. See Arthur W. Frank, *The Wounded Storyteller* (Chicago: University of Chicago Press, 1995), for an explanation of the difference between a recovery and a chaos narrative.

4. Dave Eggers, *A Heartbreaking Work of Staggering Genius* (New York: Simon and Schuster, 2000).

5. Paul John Eakin, *Living Autobiographically: How We Create Identity in Narrative* (Ithaca: Cornell University Press, 2008), 32.

6. Dwight Fee, *Pathology and the Postmodern: Mental Illness As Discourse and Experience*, ed. Dwight Fee (London: Sage Publications, 2000), 96.

7. Ibid., 3.

8. Michel Foucault, *History of Madness*, ed. Jean Khalfa, trans. Jonathan Murphy and Jean Khalfa (London: Routledge, 2006), xxvii.

9. Eakin, *Living Autobiographically*, 32.

10. Lizzie Simon, *Detour: My Bipolar Road Trip in 4-D* (New York: Washington Square Press, 2002), 210, 211.

11. Mike Barnes, *The Lily Pond: A Memoir of Madness, Memory, Myth, and Metamorphosis (Emeryville, Ont.*: Biblioasis, 2008), 75. Succeeding references to this work are cited by page number in the text.

12. Behrman, *Electroboy*, 257.

13. Lisa Diedrich, *Treatments: Language, Politics, and the Culture of Illness* (Minneapolis: University of Minnesota Press, 2007), 45.

14. Dwight Fee, "The Project of Pathology: Reflexivity and Depression in Elizabeth Wurtzel's *Prozac Nation*," in *Pathology and the Postmodern: Mental Illness As Discourse and Experience*, ed. Dwight Fee (London: Sage Publications, 2000), 96.

15. Simon, *Detour*, 209.

16. Keith Alan Steadman, *The Bipolar Expeditionist* (Bloomington, Ind.: iUniverse, 2008), 14.

17. Holly Hollan, *Soaring and Crashing: My Bipolar Adventures* (Minneapolis: Mills City Press, 2007), 109.

18. Mark Pollard, *In Small Doses: A Memoir about Accepting and Living with Bipolar Disorder* (Chicago: Near North Press, 2003), 31.

19. Ibid., 32.

20. Steadman, *Bipolar Expeditionist*, 353.

21. Hollan, *Soaring and Crashing*, 236.

22. Pollard, *In Small Doses*, 89.

23. John Forkasdi, *The Secrets Within: A Memoir of a Bipolar Man* (Tucson: Wheatmark, 2008), 59.

24. Donald Kern, *Mind Gone Awry* (Los Angeles: Isaac Nathan, 2008), 17.

25. Ibid., 69, 17.

26. Christopher Palmer, *The River Manic* (West Conshohocken, Pa.: Infinity, 2008), 62.

27. Terri Cheney, *Manic: A Memoir* (New York: HarperCollins, 2008), 61, 129.

28. Palmer, *The River Manic*, 327, 215.

29. Kern, *Mind Gone Awry*, 95.

30. Cheney, *Manic*, 184.

31. Marya Hornbacher, *Madness: A Bipolar Life* (Boston: Houghton Mifflin, 2008), 259. Succeeding references to this work are cited by page number in the text.

32. Barnes, *The Lily Pond*, 42, 188.

33. Behrman, *Electroboy*, 46. Succeeding references to this work are cited by page number in the text.

34. Cheney, *Manic*, 67.

35. Melody Hope, *In My Head: Living My Life with Bi-Polar* (Bloomington, Ind.: Xlibris, 2008), 36, 163.

36. Jane Thompson, *Sugar and Salt: My Life with Bipolar Disorder* (Bloomington, Ind.: Authorhouse, 2006), 108, 136.

37. Hollan, *Soaring and Crashing*, 182, 231.

38. Hornbacher, *Madness*, 67.

39. Kern, *Mind Gone Awry*, 19.

40. Ibid., 37.

41. Hope, *In My Head*, 89.

42. Barnes, *The Lily Pond*, 34.

43. Steadman, *Bipolar Expeditionist*, 190.

44. Simon, *Detour*, 27.

45. Thompson, *Sugar and Salt*, 129.

46. Hollan, *Soaring and Crashing*, 248, 249.

47. Ibid., 234.

48. Hornbacher, *Madness*, 275.

49. Ibid., 154, 155.

50. Steadman, *Bipolar Expeditionist*, 17.

51. Ibid., 352, 296.

52. Pollard, *In Small Doses*, 98.

53. Simon, *Detour*, 11, 22.

54. Hollan, *Soaring and Crashing*, 211, 183.

55. Hornbacher, *Madness*, 32. Succeeding references to this work are cited by page number in the text.

56. Hope, *In My Head*, 88, 106.

57. Thompson, *Sugar and Salt*, 117.

58. Forkasdi, *The Secrets Within*, 50.

59. Suzy Johnston, *The Naked Birdwatcher* (Helensburgh, U.K.: The Cairn, 2002), 53.

60. Ibid., 59.

61. Hope, *In My Head*, 36.

62. Forkasdi, *The Secrets Within*, 20.

63. Palmer, *The River Manic*, 142.

64. Cheney, *Manic*, 84. Succeeding references to this work are cited by page number in the text.

65. Kay R. Jamison, *An Unquiet Mind* (New York: Knopf, 1995), 75.

CHAPTER 5 — NEUROPSYCHIATRY, PHARMACOLOGY,
AND IMAGING THE NEW MANIA

1. Andy Clark, *Natural-born Cyborgs: Minds, Technologies, and the Future of Human Intelligence* (Oxford: Oxford University Press, 2003); Ray Kurzweil, *The Singularity Is Near: When Humans Transcend Biology* (New York: Viking, 2005).

2. Roberto B. Sassi and Jair C. Soares, "Brain Imaging Methods in Neuropsychiatry," in *Brain Imaging in Affective Disorders*, ed. Jair Soares (New York: M. Dekker, 2003), 2.

3. In *Brain Imaging in Affective Disorders*, ed. Jair Soares, (New York: M. Dekker, 2003), see, e.g., Warren D. Taylor and Ranga R. Krishnan, "Structural Brain Investigations in Affective Disorders," 53–78; Andrea L. Malizia and David J. Nutt, "Human Brain Imaging in the Development of Psychotropics: Focus on Affective and Anxiety Disorders," 321–336; Gwenn S. Smith, Kimberly Robeson, M. Elizabeth Sublette, and Bruce G. Pollock, "Positron Emission Tomography and Single Photon Emission Computed Tomography Imaging of Antidepressant Treatment Effects in Major Depression," 283–319.

4. Malizia and Nutt, "Human Brain," 334.

5. Nancy C. Andreasen, *Brave New Brain: Conquering Mental Illness in the Era of the Genome* (Oxford: Oxford University Press, 2001), 132.

6. Francis Fukuyama, *Our Posthuman Future: Consequences of the Biotechnology Revolution* (New York: Picador, 2002), 42.

7. Peter R. Breggin, *Brain-disabling Treatments in Psychiatry: Drugs, Electroshock, and the Psychopharmaceutical Complex*, 2d ed., rev. (New York: Springer, 2008), 215.

8. Fukuyama, *Our Posthuman Future*, 218.

9. Ibid., 7.

10. Soares, *Brain Imaging in Affective Disorders*, v.

11. Bettyann Holtzman Kevles, *Naked to the Bone: Medical Imaging in the Twentieth Century* (New Brunswick, N.J.: Rutgers University Press, 1997), 298.

12. Stuart C. Yudofsky and Robert E. Hales, *Essentials of Neuropsychiatry and Clinical Neurosciences*, 4th ed. (Washington, D.C.: American Psychiatric Publishing, 2004).

13. Lori L. Altshuler, Susan Y. Bookheimer, Jennifer Townsend, Manuel A. Proenza, Naomi Eisenberger, Fred Sabb, Jim Mintz, and Mark S. Cohen, "Blunted Activation in Orbitofrontal Cortex during Mania: A Functioning Magnetic Resonance Imaging Study," *Biological Psychiatry* 58 (2005): 763.

14. Roberto B. Sassi, Paolo Brambilla, John P. Hatch, Mark A. Nicoletti, Alan G. Mallinger, Ellen Frank, David J. Kupfer, Matcheri S. Keshavan, and Jair C. Soares, "Reduced Left Anterior Cingulate Volumes in Untreated Bipolar Patients," *Biological Psychiatry* 56 (2004): 468.

15. Hillary P. Blumberg, Emily Stern, Diana Martinez, Sally Ricketts, Jose de Asis, Thomas White, Jane Epstein, P. Anne McBride, David Eidelberg, James H. Kocsis, et al., "Increased Anterior Cingulate and Caudate Activity in Bipolar Mania," *Biographical Psychiatry* 48 (2000): 1045.

16. Lara C. Foland, Lori L Altshuler, Susan Y. Bookheimer, Naomi Eisenberger, Jenifer Townsend, and Paul M. Thompson, "Evidence for Deficient Modulation of Amygdala Response by Prefrontal Cortex in Bipolar Mania," *Psychiatry Research: Neuroimaging* 162 (2008): 27.

17. Sassi et al., "Reduced Left Anterior."

18. Ibid.; John O. Brooks III, "Metabolic Evidence of Corticolimbic Dysregulation in Bipolar Mania," *Psychiatry Research: Neuroimaging* 181 (2010): 137.

19. Andreasen, *Brave New Brain*, 32.

20. Joseph Dumit, *Picturing Personhood: Brain Scans and Biomedical Identity* (Princeton, N.J: Princeton University Press, 2004), 103.

21. David W. Loring, ed. *INS Dictionary of Neuropsychology* (New York: Oxford University Press, 1999), 102

22. The approval for lithium use in manic patients, however, was delayed when lithium chloride was used in the diets of cardiac and hypertensive patients; without monitoring, the dosage resulted in some lethal intoxications. See J. F. Cade, "Lithium Salts in the Treatment of Psychotic Excitement," *Medical Journal of Australia* 2 (1949): 349–352; and M. Schou, N. Juel-Nielsen, E. Stromgren, and H. Volby, "The Treatment of Manic Psychoses by the Administration of Lithium Salts," *Journal of Neurology, Neurosurgery, and Psychiatry* 17 (1954): 250–260.

23. Nathan S. Kline, *Depression: Its Diagnosis and Treatment. Lithium: The History of Its Use in Psychiatry* (New York: Brunner/Mazel, 1969), 79–80.

24. Breggin, *Brain-Disabling Treatments*, xviii. Succeeding references to this work are cited by page number in the text.

25. Brian Kean, "The Psychopharmaceutical Complex," in *Forensic Psychiatry: Influences of Evil*, ed. Tom Mason (Totowa, N.J.: Human Press, 2006), 31. Curiously, given Kean's accord with Breggin's position, Kean cites Foucault to criticize the psychiatric medical model; yet Foucault in *History of Madness* suggests that Tuke and the discourse of moral therapy are partly responsible for creating a medical model and suggests that psychotherapy has created the kind of controlling gaze that makes humans objects of scientific objectivity.

26. David Healy, *Mania: A Short History of Bipolar Disorder* (Baltimore: Johns Hopkins University Press, 2008), 100.

27. David L. Herzberg, *From Miltown to Prozac: Happy Pills in America* (Baltimore: Johns Hopkins University Press, 2009), 150–191.

28. J. J. Schildkraut, "Neuropsychopharmacology and the Affective Disorders (First of Three Parts)," *New England Journal of Medicine* 4 (1969): 197–201.

29. J. J. Schildkraut, "Neuropsychopharmacology and the Affective Disorders (Third of Three Parts)," *New England Journal of Medicine* 6 (1969): 302–308.

30. Clark, *Natural-born Cyborgs*, 194.

31. Nikolas Rose, *The Politics of Life Itself: Biomedicine, Power, and Subjectivity in the Twenty-First Century* (Princeton, N.J.: Princeton University Press, 2006), 188.

32. Andrew Lakoff, *Pharmaceutical Reason: Knowledge and Value in Global Psychiatry* (New York: Cambridge University Press, 2005), 176.

EPILOGUE

1. Edward Shorter, *A History of Psychiatry: From the Era of the Asylum to the Age of Prozac* (New York: John Wiley and Sons, 1997), 114.

2. S. Weir Mitchell, *Wear and Tear; or, Hints for the Overworked* (Philadelphia: J. B. Lippincott, 1899).

3. Michael J. Clark, "Anxiety Disorders: Social Section," in *A History of Clinical Psychiatry: The Origin and History of Psychiatric Disorders*, ed. German E. Berrios and Roy Porter (New Brunswick, N.J.: Athlone Press, 1995), 563–572.

4. Ibid., 568, 569.

5. Ibid., 415.

6. Jackie Orr, *Panic Diaries: A Genealogy of Panic Disorder* (Durham, N.C.: Duke University Press, 2006), 9.

7. Ibid., 280; Clark, "Anxiety," 565; David Healy, *Mania: A Short History of Bipolar Disorder* (Baltimore: Johns Hopkins University Press, 2008), 66.

8. Peter C. Whybrow, *American Mania: When More Is Not Enough* (New York: Norton, 2005), 4.

9. John D. Gartner, *The Hypomanic Edge: The Link between Craziness and Success in America* (New York Simon and Schuster, 2005), 7.

10. Ibid., 11.

11. Emily Martin, *Bipolar Expeditions: Mania and Depression in American Culture* (Princeton, N.J.: Princeton University Press, 2007), 220.

12. Data drawn from Stephen Jones and Richard Bentall, "Introductory Overview," *The Psychology of Bipolar Disorder* (Oxford: Oxford University Press, 2006), 1–2.

13. National Alliance for Mental Illness, http://www.nami.org/.

14. Films Media Group, *The Medicated Child* (2008), http://stats.lib.pdx.edu/proxy.php?url=http://digital.films.com/play/A9KJDM.

15. Dana H. Perry, Hart Perry, and Michael Bacon, *Boy Interrupted* (HBO Documentary Films, 2009).

16. American Psychiatric Association, "Report of the DSM-V Childhood and Adolescent Disorders Work Group," http://www.psych.org/MainMenu/Research/DSMIV/DSMV/DSMRevisionActivities/DSM-V-Work-Group-Reports/Childhood-and-Adolescent-Disorders-Work-Group-Report.aspx.

17. Ibid.

18. The Child and Adolescent Bipolar Foundation, "Parents of Bipolar Children Applaud New DSM-V Diagnostic Category, but Call for a More Accurate Name" (February 18, 2010), http://www.bpkids.org/about/press/dsm-v?utm_source=Child+and+Adolescent+Bipolar+Foundation+Listandutm_campaign=be155cf63c-DSM_2_26_2010 andutm_medium=email.

BIBLIOGRAPHY

Akiskal, Hagop S. "The Prevalent Clinical Spectrum of Bipolar Disorders: Beyond DSM-IV." *Journal of Clinical Psychopharmacology* 62 (1996): 4S–14S.

Akiskal, Hagop S., Marc L. Bourgeois, Jules Angst, Robert Post, Hans-Jürgen Möller, and Robert Hirschfeld. "Re-Evaluating the Prevalence of and Diagnostic Composition within the Broad Clinical Spectrum of Bipolar Disorders." *Journal of Affective Disorders* 59 (2000): S5–S30.

Alda, Martin. "In Memoriam: Professor George Winokur." *Journal of Psychiatry and Neuroscience* 22.1 (January 1997): 70.

Altshuler, Lori L., Susan Y. Bookheimer, Jennifer Townsend, Manuel A. Proenza, Naomi Eisenberger, Fred Sabb, Jim Mintz, and Mark S. Cohen. "Blunted Activation in Orbitofrontal Cortex during Mania: A Functioning Magnetic Resonance Imaging Study." *Biological Psychiatry* 58 (2005): 763–769.

American Psychiatric Association. *Diagnostic and Statistical Manual of Mental Disorders: DSM-IV-TR*. Washington, D.C.: American Psychiatric Association, 2000.

Andreasen, Nancy C. *Brave New Brain: Conquering Mental Illness in the Era of the Genome*. Oxford: Oxford University Press, 2001.

Appeal to the People of Pennsylvania on the Subject of an Asylum for the Insane Poor. Philadelphia: Printed for the Committee, 1838.

Aurelianus, Caelius. "Madness or Insanity (Greek: Mania)." In *Documentary History of Psychiatry*, ed. Charles E. Goshen, 18–31. New York: Philosophical Library, 1967.

Baethge, Christopher, Paula Salvorte, and Ross J. Baldessarini. "'On Cyclic Insanity' by Karl Ludwig Kahlbaum MD: A Translation and Commentary." *Harvard Review of Psychiatry* (March/April 2003): 78–90.

Barnes, Mike. *The Lily Pond: A Memoir of Madness, Memory, Myth, and Metamorphosis*. Emeryville, Ont.: Biblioasis, 2008.

Barondes, Samuel H. *Better Than Prozac: Creating the Next Generation of Psychiatric Drugs*. New York: Oxford University Press, 2003.

Baszanger, Isabelle. *Inventing Pain Medicine: From the Laboratory to the Clinic*. New Brunswick, N.J.: Rutgers University Press, 1998.

Baudrillard, Jean. *Forget Foucault*. Edited by Sylvère Lotringer. Translated by Nicole Dufresne. Los Angeles: Semiotext, 2007. First published 1970 by Small Press.

Behrman, Andy. *Electroboy: A Memoir of Mania.* New York: Random House, 2002.

Berg, Marc, and Annemarie Mol. *Differences in Medicine: Unraveling Practices, Techniques, and Bodies.* Durham, N.C: Duke University Press, 1998.

Berrios, G. E. "Classic Text No. 57: Of Mania: (from Bucknill and Tuke, 1858)." *History of Psychiatry* 15.1 (2004): 105–111.

———. "Mood Disorders." In *A History of Clinical Psychiatry: The Origin and History of Psychiatric Disorders,* ed. German Berrios and Roy Porter, 384–408. London: Athlone Press, 1995.

Biagioli, Mario, and Peter Galison. *Scientific Authorship: Credit and Intellectual Property in Science.* New York: Routledge, 2003.

Blackburn, Isaac Wright. *Illustrations of the Gross Morbid Anatomy of the Brain in the Insane.* Washington, D.C.: Government Printing Office, 1908.

Blumberg, Hillary P., Emily Stern, Diana Martinez, Sally Ricketts, Jose de Asis, Thomas White, Jane Epstein, P. Anne McBride, David Eidelberg, James H. Kocsis, et al. "Increased Anterior Cingulate and Caudate Activity in Bipolar Mania." *Biological Psychiatry* 48 (2000): 1045–1052.

Boerhaave, Herman. "Of the Maniacal or Roving Madness." In *Documentary History of Psychiatry,* ed. Charles Goshen, 228–240. New York: Philosophical Library, 1967.

Boston Lunatic Hospital. *Report of the Superintendent of the Boston Lunatic Hospital and Physician of the Public Institution at South Boston.* Boston: John H. Eastburn, 1840.

Bowers, Len. *The Social Nature of Mental Illness.* New York: Routledge, 1998.

Breggin, Peter R. *Brain-Disabling Treatments in Psychiatry: Drugs, Electroshock, and the Psychopharmaceutical Complex.* 2d edition, revised. New York: Springer, 2008.

Brooks, John O., III. "Metabolic Evidence of Cortocolimbic Dysregulation in Bipolar Mania." *Psychiatry Research: Neuroimaging* 181 (2010): 136–140.

Bucknill, John Charles, and Daniel Hack Tuke. *A Manual of Psychological Medicine.* 3d ed. Philadelphia: Lindsay and Blakiston, 1874.

Castle, Lana R. *Finding Your Bipolar Muse: How to Master Depressive Droughts and Manic Floods and Access Your Creative Power.* New York: Marlowe, 2006.

Cheney, Terri. *Manic: A Memoir.* New York: HarperCollins, 2008.

Chesler, Phyllis. *Women and Madness.* New York: Avon, 1972.

Clark, Andy. *Natural-born Cyborgs: Minds, Technologies, and the Future of Human Intelligence.* Oxford: Oxford University Press, 2003.

Clark, Michael J. "Anxiety Disorders: Social Section." In *A History of Clinical Psychiatry: The Origin and History of Psychiatric Disorders,* ed. German E. Berrios and Roy Porter, 563–572. New Brunswick, N.J.: Athlone Press, 1995.

Conrad, Peter, and Joseph W. Schneider. *Deviance and Medicalization: From Badness to Sickness.* Reprinted with a new afterword by the authors. Philadelphia: Temple University Press, 1992. First published 1980 by C. V. Mosby, St. Louis.

Contributors to the Asylum for the Relief of Persons Deprived of the Use of Their Reason. *Annual Report on the State of the Asylum for the Relief of Persons Derived of the Use of Their Reason.* Philadelphia: Philadelphia Asylum, 1835.

———. *Annual Report on the State of the Asylum for the Relief of Persons Derived of the Use of Their Reason.* Philadelphia: Philadelphia Asylum, 1838.

Cullen, William. *First Lines of the Practice of Physic.* Vol. 4. Edinburgh: C. Elliot, 1784.

Daston, Lorraine, ed. *Biographies of Scientific Objects.* Chicago: University of Chicago Press, 2000.

Denning, Michael. *Mechanic Accents: Dime Novels and Working-Class Culture in America.* New York: Verso, 1987.

Deutsch, Albert. *The Mentally Ill in America: A History of Their Care and Treatment from Colonial Times.* New York: Columbia University Press, 1949.

Dickens, Charles. *American Notes for General Circulation.* Edited by Patricia Ingham. New York: Penguin Classics, 1985.

Diedrich, Lisa. *Treatments: Language, Politics, and the Culture of Illness.* Minneapolis: University of Minnesota Press, 2007.

Diethelm, O. "Mania: A Clinical Study of Dissertations before 1750." *Confinia Psychiatrica* 13.9 (1970): 26–49.

Dix, Dorothea L. *Memorial to the Legislature of Massachusetts.* Lyrasis Members and Sloan Foundation, 2009. First printed 1843 by Munroe and Francis, Boston. http://www .archive.org/details/memorialtolegis100dixd.

Duganne, A.J.H. *The Knights of the Seal; or, The Mysteries of the Three Cities: A Romance of Men's Hearts and Habits.* Philadelphia: Colon and Adriance, 1845.

Duke, Patty, and Gloria Hochman. *A Brilliant Madness: Living with Manic-Depressive Illness.* New York: Bantam Books, 1992.

Dumit, Joseph. *Picturing Personhood: Brain Scans and Biomedical Identity.* Princeton, N.J.: Princeton University Press, 2004.

Dunner, D. L. "Clinical Consequences of Under-Recognized Bipolar Spectrum Disorder." *Bipolar Disorder* 5 (2003): 456–463.

Dunner, D. L., E. S. Gershon, and F. K. Goodwin. "Heritable Factors in the Severity of Affective Illnesses." *Scientific Proceedings, American Psychiatric Association* 123 (1970): 187–188.

Eakin, Paul John. *Living Autobiographically: How We Create Identity in Narrative.* Ithaca: Cornell University Press, 2008.

Eastern Lunatic Asylum. *Report of the Eastern Lunatic Asylum: In the City of Williamsburg, Virginia, 1851.* Richmond: Ritchies and Dunnavant, 1852.

———. *Report of the Eastern Lunatic Asylum: In the City of Williamsburg, Virginia, 1856.* Richmond: Ritchies and Dunnavant, 1857.

Eggers, Dave. *A Heartbreaking Work of Staggering Genius.* New York: Simon and Schuster, 2000.

Erickson, Paul Joseph. "Welcome to Sodom: The Cultural Work of City-Mysteries Fiction in Antebellum America." PhD diss. University of Texas at Austin, 2005.

Esquirol, Etienne. *Mental Maladies: A Treatise on Insanity.* Philadelphia: Lee and Blanchard, 1845.

Fee, Dwight. *Pathology and the Postmodern: Mental Illness As Discourse and Experience.* London: Sage Publications, 2000.

Fieve, Ronald R. *Bipolar II: Enhance Your Highs, Boost Your Creativity, and Escape the Cycles of Recurrent Depression: The Essential Guide to Recognize and Treat the Mood Swings of This Increasingly Common Disorder.* New York: Rodale, 2006.

Foland, Lara C., Lori L Altshuler, Susan Y. Bookheimer, Naomi Eisenberger, Jenifer Townsend, and Paul M. Thompson. "Evidence for Deficient Modulation of Amygdala Response by Prefrontal Cortex in Bipolar Mania." *Psychiatry Research: Neuroimaging* 162 (2008): 27–37.

Forkasdi, John C. *The Secrets Within: A Memoir of a Bipolar Man.* Tucson: Wheatmark, 2008.

Foucault, Michel. *History of Madness.* Edited by Jean Khalfa. Translated by Jonathan Murphy and Jean Khalfa. Foreword by Ian Hacking. London: Routledge, 2006.

———. *Psychiatric Power: Lectures at the College de France, 1973–1974.* Edited by Jacques Lagrange. Translated by Graham Burchell. New York: Picador, 2008.

Frank, Arthur W. *The Wounded Storyteller.* Chicago: University of Chicago Press, 1995.

Freedman, Alfred M., Harold I. Kaplan, and Benjamin J. Sadock. *Comprehensive Textbook of Psychiatry, II.* Baltimore: Williams and Wilkins, 1975.

Freud, Sigmund. "Mourning and Melancholia." In *Standard Edition of the Complete Psychological Works of Sigmund Freud.* Vol. 14. Edited and translated by James Strachey. London: Hogarth Press, 1957.

Fukuyama, Francis. *Our Posthuman Future.* London: Profile, 2007.

Gartner, John D. *The Hypomanic Edge: The Link between Craziness and Success in America.* New York: Simon and Schuster, 2005.

Gauchet, Marcel, and Gladys Swain. *Madness and Democracy: The Modern Psychiatric Universe.* Princeton, N.J.: Princeton University Press, 1999.

Gelder, Michael, Nancy Andreasen, Juan Lopez-Ibor, and John Geddes, eds., *New Oxford Textbook of Psychiatry,* 2d ed. (Oxford: Oxford University Press, 2009).

Goffman, Erving. *Asylums: Essays on the Social Situation of Mental Patients and Other Inmates.* Garden City, N.Y.: Anchor, 1961.

Goodwin, Guy. "Hypomania: What's in a Name?" Editorial. *British Journal of Psychiatry* 181 (2002): 94–95.

Goshen, Charles E., ed. *Documentary History of Psychiatry.* New York: Philosophical Library, 1967.

Grob, Gerald N. *Mental Institutions in America: Social Policy to 1875.* New York: Free Press, 1973.

"Gulltown in an Uproar!!" Cartoon. Philadelphia: J. L. Magee, c. 1865.

Hacking, Ian. *Historical Ontology.* Cambridge, Mass.: Harvard University Press, 2002.

Hall, David D. *Cultures of Print: Essays in the History of the Book.* Amherst: University of Massachusetts Press, 1996.

Hare, Edward. "The Two Manias: A Study of the Evolution of the Modern Concept of Mania." *British Journal of Psychiatry* 138 (1981): 89–99.

Hare, Samuel. *Statistical Report of One Hundred and Ninety Cases of Insanity, Admitted into the Retreat, near Leeds.* London: S. Taylor, printer, 1843.

Healy, David. *Let Them Eat Prozac: The Unhealthy Relationship between the Pharmaceutical Industry and Depression.* New York: New York University Press, 2004.

———. *Mania: A Short History of Bipolar Disorder.* Baltimore: Johns Hopkins University Press, 2008.

Hecker, J.F.C. *The Dancing Mania of the Middle Ages.* New York: Burt Franklin, 1837.

Herzberg, David L. *Happy Pills in America: From Miltown to Prozac.* Baltimore: Johns Hopkins University Press, 2009.

Hill, Gershom H. "Prognosis in Insanity." *Iowa Medical Journal* (October 1895): 379–382.

Hollan, Holly. *Soaring and Crashing: My Bipolar Adventures.* Minneapolis: Mills City Press, 2007.

Hope, Melody. *In My Head: Living My Life with Bi-Polar.* Bloomington, Ind.: Xlibris, 2008.

Hornbacher, Marya. *Madness: A Bipolar Life.* Boston: Houghton Mifflin, 2008.

Hospital for the Insane at Independence. *First Biennial Report of the Hospital for the Insane at Independence.* Des Moines: Hospital for the Insane at Independence, 1874.

Howe, Daniel Walker. *What Hath God Wrought: The Transformation of America, 1815–1848.* New York: Oxford University Press, 2007.

Illinois State Hospital for the Insane. *Ninth Biennial Report of the Trustees, Superintendent and Treasurer of the Illinois State Hospital for the Insane at Jacksonville.* Springfield, Ill.: Baker and Phillips, printers, 1864.

Iowa Board of Control of State Institutions. *Biennial Report of the Board of Control of State Institutions of Iowa*. Des Moines: State printer, June 1914.

———. *State of Iowa Bulletin of State Institutions*. Anamosa, Iowa: Reformatory Press, 1922.

Iowa Hospital for the Insane. *Report of the Officers of the Iowa Hospital for the Insane to the Governor of the State of Iowa: For the Fiscal Years 1866–67*. Des Moines: F. W. Palmer, state printer, 1868.

Jamison, Kay R. *An Unquiet Mind*. New York: Knopf, 1995.

Johnston, Suzy. *The Naked Birdwatcher*. Helensburgh, U.K.: The Cairn, 2002.

Joint Committee of Council and Assembly, Trenton. *Report Relative to an Asylum for Lunatics, by the Joint Committee of Council and Assembly*. Trenton, N.J.: Sherman and Harron, 1841.

Jones, Stephen, and Richard Bentall. "Introductory Overview." The Psychology of Bipolar Disorder. Oxford: Oxford University Press, 2006.

Kean, Brian. "The Psychopharmaceutical Complex." In *Forensic Psychiatry: Influences of Evil*, ed. Tom Mason, 31–65. Totowa, N.J.: Humana Press, 2006.

Kern, Donald. *Mind Gone Awry*. Los Angeles: Isaac Nathan, 2008.

Kevles, Bettyann Holtzman. *Naked to the Bone: Medical Imaging in the Twentieth Century*. New Brunswick, N.J: Rutgers University Press, 1997.

Klerman, G. L. "The Spectrum of Mania." *Comprehensive Psychiatry* 22 (1981): 11–20.

Kline, Nathan S. *Depression: Its Diagnosis and Treatment. Lithium: The History of Its Use in Psychiatry*. New York: Brunner/Mazel, 1969.

Kotsopoulos, Sotiris. "Aretaeus the Cappadocian on Mental Illness." *Comprehensive Psychiatry* 27.2 (1986): 171–179.

Kraepelin, Emil. *Manic Depressive Insanity and Paranoia*. Edinburgh: Livingstone, 1921; reprinted in *Manic-depressive Illness: History of a Syndrome*, ed. Edward A. Wolpert, 33–114. New York: International Universities Press, 1977. References are to the 1977 reprint.

Kraepelin, Emil, and A. R. Diefendorf. *Clinical Psychiatry: A Text-Book for Students and Physicians*. In *Lifetime Editions of Kraepelin in English*. Vol. 2. Bristol: Thoemmes Press, 2002.

Kramer, Peter D. *Listening to Prozac*. New York: Penguin Books, 1997.

Kurzweil, Ray. *The Singularity Is Near: When Humans Transcend Biology*. New York: Viking, 2005.

Lakoff, Andrew. *Pharmaceutical Reason: Knowledge and Value in Global Psychiatry*. New York: Cambridge University Press, 2005.

Latour, Bruno. *Pandora's Hope: Essays on the Reality of Science Studies*. New York: Cambridge University Press. 1999.

Law, John. *After Method: Mess in Social Science Research*. London: Routledge, 2004.

Law, John, and Annemarie Mol, eds. *Complexities: Social Studies of Knowledge Practices*. Durham, N.C.: Duke University Press, 2002.

Law, John, and Vicky Singleton. "Performing Technology's Stories: On Social Constructivism, Performance, and Performativity." *Technology and Culture* 41.4 (2000): 765–775.

Loring, David, ed. *INS Dictionary of Neuropsychiatry*. New York: Oxford University Press, 1999.

Lunatic Asylum of South Carolina. *Lunatic Asylum of South Carolina: Report of the Committee of Regents, Report of the Physician, Report of the Superintendent, Laws of the Institution, etc.* Columbia: Morgan Isaac, 1842.

Martin, Emily. *Bipolar Expeditions: Mania and Depression in American Culture.* Princeton, N.J.: Princeton University Press, 2007.

Maudsley, Henry. "Edgar Allen Poe." *Journal of Insanity* 17.2 (October 1860): 153–198.

Metzel, Jonathan. *Prozac on the Couch: Prescribing Gender in the Era of Wonder Drugs.* Durham, N.C.: Duke University Press, 2003.

M'Gugin, D. L. "Cases in Practice." *Iowa Medical Journal,* August/September 1855, 179–182.

———. "Outraged Laws of Hygiene." *Iowa Medical Journal,* June/July 1855, 407–413.

Mitchell, S. Weir. *Wear and Tear; or, Hints for the Overworked.* Philadelphia: J. B. Lippincott, 1899.

Mol, Annemarie. *The Body Multiple: Ontology in Medical Practice.* Durham, N.C.: Duke University Press, 2002.

"Money-Making Mania." Editorial. *Journal of Insanity,* April 1849, 327–343.

Müller-Wille, Staffan, and Hans-Jörg Rheinberger. *Heredity Produced: At the Crossroads of Biology, Politics, and Culture, 1500–1870.* Cambridge, Mass: MIT Press, 2007.

Munchausen, Philosopher's Stone, and Gull Creek Grand Consolidated Oil Company. Prospectus. Pittsburgh: John W. Pittock, c. 1865.

National Alliance for Mental Illness. http://www.nami.org/.

New Hampshire Asylum for the Insane/George Chandler. *Reports of the Board of Visitors, of the Trustees, and of the Superintendent of the New Hampshire Asylum for the Insane: June Session, 1843.* Concord, N.H.: Carroll and Baker, 1843.

New Jersey State Lunatic Asylum. *Report of the Managers of the New Jersey State Lunatic Asylum.* Trenton: n.p., 1854.

New York State Lunatic Asylum. *Annual Report of the Managers of the New York State Lunatic Asylum.* 1844.

———. *Thirteenth Annual Report of the Managers of the New York State Lunatic Asylum.* Albany: C. Van Benthuysen, printer to the Legislature, 1856.

———. *Thirty-First Annual Report of the Managers of the New York State Lunatic Asylum.* Albany: Weed, Parsons, printers, 1873.

Ohio Lunatic Asylum. *Annual Report of the Directors of the Ohio Lunatic Asylum.* Columbus: Samuel Medary, 1839.

———. *Third Annual Report of the Directors of the Ohio Lunatic Asylum.* Columbus: n.p., 1837.

Orr, Jackie. *Panic Diaries: A Genealogy of Panic Disorder.* Durham, N.C.: Duke University Press, 2006.

Palmer, Christopher. *The River Manic.* West Conshohocken, Pa.: Infinity, 2008.

Paracelsus. "Diseases That Deprive Man of His Reason." In *Documentary History of Psychiatry,* ed. Charles Goshen. New York: Philosophical Library, 1967.

Pargeter, William. *Observations on Maniacal Disorders.* Edited with a foreword by Stanley W. Jackson. London: Routledge, 1988. First published 1792.

"Patients, Admissions, etc., 1752–1786." Archives of the Pennsylvania Hospital, Philadelphia.

Pauley, Jane. *Skywriting: A Life out of the Blue.* New York: Random House, 2004.

Pennsylvania Hospital. *Annual Report of the Department for the Insane of the Pennsylvania Hospital.* Philadelphia: Press of Lehman and Bolton, 1891.

———. *Annual Report of the Department for the Insane of the Pennsylvania Hospital.* Philadelphia: n.p., 1896.

———. *Report of the Board of Managers of the Pennsylvania Hospital.* Philadelphia: Collins, 1886.

———. *Report of the Pennsylvania Hospital for the Insane for the Year 1883*. Philadelphia: n.p., 1884.

Pennsylvania Hospital for the Insane. *Annual Report of the Pennsylvania Hospital for the Insane*. Philadelphia: T. K. and P. G. Collins, printers, 1856.

———. *Report of the Pennsylvania Hospital for the Insane*. Philadelphia: James C. Haswell, printers, 1842.

———. *Report of the Pennsylvania Hospital for the Insane*. Philadelphia: T. K. and P. G. Collins, printers, 1860.

———. *Report of the Pennsylvania Hospital for the Insane for the Year 1882*. Philadelphia: T. K. and P. G. Collins, printers, 1883.

Pinel, Philippe. *A Treatise on Insanity: In Which Are Contained the Principles of a New and More Practical Nosology of Maniacal Disorders Than Has Yet Been Offered to the Public*. Translated by D. D. Davis. The Strand, London: W. Todd for Cadell and Davies, 1806.

Poe, Edgar Allan. "The System of Doctor Tarr and Professor Fether." 1845. Baltimore: Edgar Allan Poe Society of Baltimore. http://www.eapoe.org/works/tales/tarrb.htm.

Pollard, Marc. *In Small Doses: A Memoir about Accepting and Living with Bipolar Disorder*. Chicago: Near North Press, 2003.

Reiss, Benjamin. *Theaters of Madness: Insane Asylums and Nineteenth-Century American Culture*. Chicago: University of Chicago Press, 2008.

Report of the Proceedings for Establishing a Board of Commissioners in Lunacy for the State of New York. New York: A. G. Sherwood, 1880.

Reynolds, David S. *Beneath the American Renaissance: The Subversive Imagination in the Age of Emerson and Melville*. Cambridge, Mass.: Harvard University Press, 1988.

Rose, Nikolas. *The Politics of Life Itself: Biomedicine, Power, and Subjectivity in the Twenty-First Century*. Princeton, N.J.: Princeton University Press, 2006.

Rothman, David J. *The Discovery of the Asylum: Social Order and Disorder in the New Republic*. Boston: Little, Brown, 1971.

Sadock, Benjamin J., and Virginia A. Sadock. *Comprehensive Textbook of Psychiatry*. Philadelphia: Lippincott Williams and Wilkins, 2000.

Sassi, Roberto B., Paolo Brambilla, John P. Hatch, Mark A. Nicoletti, Alan G. Mallinger, Ellen Frank, David J. Kupfer, Matcheri S. Keshavan, and Jair C. Soares. "Reduced Left Anterior Cingulate Volumes in Untreated Bipolar Patients." *Biological Psychiatry* 56 (2004): 467–475.

Sassi. Roberto B., and Jair C. Soares. "Brain Imaging Methods in Neuropsychiatry." In *Brain Imaging in Affective Disorders*, ed. Jair C. Soares. New York: M. Dekker, 2003.

Schildkraut, J. J. "Neuropsychopharmacology and the Affective Disorders (First of Three Parts)." *New England Journal of Medicine* 281.4 (1969): 197–201.

———. "Neuropsychopharmacology and the Affective Disorders (Third of Three Parts)." *New England Journal of Medicine* 281.6 (1969): 302–308.

Scull, Andrew T. *The Museums of Madness: The Social Organization of Madness in Nineteenth-Century England*. London: St. Martin's Press, 1979.

———. *Social Order/Mental Disorder: Anglo-American Psychiatry in Historical Perspective*. Berkeley: University of California Press, 1989.

Sedler, M. J. "Falret's Discovery: The Origin of the Concept of Bipolar Affective Disorder." Translated by Mark Sedler and Eric C. Dessain. *American Journal of Psychiatry* 140.9 (September 1983): 1127–1133.

Shorter, Edward. *A History of Psychiatry: From the Era of the Asylum to the Age of Prozac*. New York: John Wiley and Sons, 1997.

Simon, Lizzie. *Detour: My Bipolar Road Trip in 4-D.* New York: Washington Square Press, 2002.

Smith, E. N., C. S. Bloss, J. A. Badner, T. Barrett, P. L. Belmonte, W. Berrettini, W. Byerley, W. Coryell, D. Craig, H. J. Edenberg, E. Eskin, et al. "Genome-wide Association Study of Bipolar Disorder in European American and African American Individuals." *Molecular Psychiatry* 14.8 (2009): 755–763.

Soares, Jair C. *Brain Imaging in Affective Disorders.* New York: M. Dekker, 2003.

State Asylum for New Jersey Lunatics. *Report of the Commissioners Appointed by the Governor of New Jersey to Ascertain the Number of Lunatics and Idiots in the State.* Newark: M. S. Harrison, 1840.

State Lunatic Hospital at Worcester. *Third Annual Report of the Trustees of the State Lunatic Hospital at Worcester.* Boston: Dutton and Wentworth, 1835.

State of New York. *Extract from the Ninth Annual Report of the State Board of Charities of the State of New York, Relating to Hospitals for the Sick and Insane.* Albany: Weed, Parsons, printers, 1876.

Steadman, Keith Alan. *The Bipolar Expeditionist.* Bloomington, Ind.: iUniverse, 2008.

Streeby, Shelley. *American Sensations: Class, Empire, and the Production of Popular Culture.* Berkeley: University of California Press, 2002.

Szasz, Thomas. *The Myth of Mental Illness: Foundations of a Theory of Personal Conduct.* New York: Harper and Row, 1961.

Tennessee Lunatic Asylum. *First Report of the Physician of the Tennessee Lunatic Asylum: To the Legislature of Tennessee, for 1840 and 1841.* Nashville: W. F. Bang, 1841.

Thompson, Charis. *Making Parents: The Ontological Choreography of Reproductive Technologies.* Cambridge, Mass.: MIT Press, 2005.

Thompson, Jane. *Sugar and Salt: My Life with Bipolar Disorder.* Bloomington, Ind.: Authorhouse, 2006.

Thurtle, Phillip. *The Emergence of Genetic Rationality: Space, Time, and Information in American Biological Science, 1870–1920.* Seattle: University of Washington Press, 2007.

Tomes, Nancy. *The Art of Asylum-Keeping: Thomas Story Kirkbride and the Origins of American Psychiatry.* Philadelphia: University of Pennsylvania Press, 1994.

Tuke, Samuel. *Description of the Retreat, an Institution near York, for Insane Persons of the Society of Friends.* Philadelphia: Isaac Pierce, 1813.

Vermont State Asylum. *Second Annual Report of the Trustees of the Vermont Asylum for the Insane, Presented to the Legislature October, 1838.* Montpelier: E. P. Walton and Son, 1838.

———. *Twenty-Fifth Annual Report of the Officers of the Vermont Asylum for the Insane.* Brattleboro: George E. Selleck, printer, 1861.

———. *Twenty-Fourth Annual Report of the Officers of the Vermont Asylum for the Insane.* Brattleboro: George E. Selleck, printer, 1860.

———. *Twenty-Seventh Annual Report of the Officers of the Vermont Asylum for the Insane.* Brattleboro: D. W. Selleck, printer, 1863.

Weiner, Debra B. "Philippe Pinel's 'Memoir on Madness' of December 11, 1794: A Fundamental Text of Modern Psychiatry." *American Journal of Psychiatry* 149.6 (1992): 725–732.

Western Lunatic Asylum. *Report of the Physician of the Western Lunatic Hospital.* Staunton, Va.: n.p., 1836.

———. *Sixteenth Annual Report of the President and Directors of the Western Lunatic Asylum, to the Legislature of Virginia: With the Report of the Superintendent and Physician, for 1842.* Staunton, Va.: Printed at the Spectator Office, 1843.

Whybrow, Peter C. *American Mania: When More Is Not Enough*. New York: Norton, 2005.

Willis, Thomas. *Dr Willis's Practice of Physick: Being the Whole Works of That Renowned and Famous Physician*. London: Printed for Dring, Harper and Leigh, 1684.

Winokur, George. *Mania and Depression: A Classification of Syndrome and Disease*. Baltimore: Johns Hopkins University Press, 1991.

Winokur, George, and Ming T. Tsuang. *The Natural History of Mania, Depression, and Schizophrenia*. Washington, D.C.: American Psychiatric Press, 1996.

Wirth-Cauchon, Janet. *Women and Borderline Personality Disorder: Symptoms and Stories*. New Brunswick, N.J.: Rutgers University Press, 2001.

Yanni, Carla. *The Architecture of Madness: Insane Asylums in the United States*. Minneapolis: University of Minnesota Press, 2007.

Yudofsky, Stuart C., and Robert E. Hales, eds. *Essentials of Neuropsychiatry and Clinical Neurosciences*. 4th ed. Washington, D.C.: American Psychiatric Publishing, 2004.

INDEX

Bolded page numbers refer to illustrations.

Abilify, 115
activity, heightened, 34–35
Acts of the Thirty-fourth General
   Assembly of Iowa (1911), 68–69
admission records, categories of insanity
   on, 42
Akiskal, H. S., 32
algorithms used in brain scans, 105
Altshuler, Lori, 103
American College of
   Neuropsychopharmacology, 111
American Mania (Whybrow), 118
American Notes (Dickens), 60, 61
American Psychiatric Association (APA),
   4, 25, 120–121
Andreasen, Nancy, 33, 99
ANK$_3$ gene, 76
*Annual Report of the Department for the
   Insane of the Pennsylvania Hospital*
   (1896), 56
*Annual Report of the Directors of the Ohio
   Lunatic Asylum* (1839), 42
*Annual Report of the Managers of the
   New York State Lunatic Asylum*
   (1844), 52
*Annual Report of the State Board of Chari-
   ties of the State of New York*
   (1876), 56
*Annual Report of the Trustees of the
   State Lunatic Hospital at Worcester*
   (1835), 50
antidepressants, 110
antipsychotics, atypical, 110
anxiety disorder, 117–118

*Appeal to the People of Pennsylvania on the
   Subject of an Asylum for the Insane Poor*
   (1838), 45
Aretaeus of Cappadocia, 2–4, 15–16, 19
Arfwedson, John, 110
Aristotelian rhetoric, 6–7
Association of Medical Superintendents
   of American Institutions for the
   Insane, 42
asylum architecture: in asylum reports, 10;
   and classes of madness, 51; detached
   structures, 47, 52, 53, 54; Kirkbride
   model, 43
asylum reform: and public opinion, 40–41;
   rhetoric of, 37–39, 58–62
asylum reports: asylum architecture in, 10;
   definitions of mania in, 37, 47; on
   heredity as cause of insanity, 67; manic
   doubling in, 48; and new democracy, 46;
   public as audience of, 44–46; statistical
   tables in, 42, 51, 67
asylums: classification of patients in, 42,
   51–54; class in, 42–43; confinement to,
   48–51, 55; custodial care in, 56, 64; deaths
   in, 56–57; early and proper treatment in,
   46, 48; literary fascination with, 62; as
   only proper place for cases of insanity,
   46–47; patient interviews in, 72–73;
   readmission to, 55–56; as symbolic of
   social reform, 61; techniques of care in, 44;
   and violent patients, 52. *See also* moral
   treatment
Auden, W. H., 117
Aurelianus, Caelius, 16

authors with mental illness, 11, 84–88.
  See also narratives, mental illness
autobiographies and autopathographies,
  82–83. *See also* narratives, mental
  illness

Barnes, Mike, 85, 88, 90
Barondes, Samuel, 112
basal ganglia chlorine, 101
Basanger, Isabelle, 9
Beard, George, 117
Behrman, Andy, 81–82, 85, 88
Berrios, German, 2
"Better Baby Contest," 69
*Better Than Prozac: Creating the Next
  Generation of Psychiatric Drugs*
  (Barondes), 112
bile, black, 16
bipolar autobiographies. *See* narratives,
  mental illness
bipolar collective, 85–86
Bipolar Consortium (Genetics Initiative
  for Bipolar Disorder Consortium), 75–76
bipolar disorder: and children, 119–121;
  first descriptions of, 23; genomic
  research on, 75–78; and heredity, 68;
  individual shape of symptomology, 86;
  and Kraepelin, 25; as a leading cause of
  disability, 119; overdiagnosis of in
  children, 120; relapses, 55–56, 119;
  spectrum of, 31, 32–34, 35. *See also*
  mania; narratives, mental illness
Bipolar Expeditionist (Steadman), 86
Bipolar Expeditions (Martin), 9
Bipolar IIB, 33
Bipolar I/II, 32
blood flow, cerebral, 102, 103
Body Multiple, The (Mol), 7
Boerhaave, Hermann, 19
Boy Interrupted (2008 film), 120
"Brain, The: the Cerebral Cortex"
  (Dryander), **106**
*Brain-Disabling Treatments in Psychiatry:
  Drugs, Electroshock, and the
  Psychopharmaceutical Complex*
  (Breggin), 111
Brain Imaging in Affective Disorders
  (Sassi and Soares), 99, 101
brain mechanisms: language of, 107; and
  mania, 35, 100; and manic markers,
  101–104; and medical technologies, 99
brain scans, 11, 101–104, 105–107, 109–110.
  See also neuroimaging technologies
Brave New Brain (Andreasen), 99
Brave New World (Huxley), 100
Breggin, Peter R., 100, 111–112

Broad Institute Center for Genotyping and
  Analysis, 78
Browers, Len, 9
Bruegel the Elder, Pieter, 17
Bucknill, John Charles, 23–24
Bulletin of State Institutions, 68

Cade, John, 111
Castle, Lana, 33
causes of insanity, 64, 67, 68
celebrities and mania, 82
chains, use of, 5, 10, 37–39, 45–46, 62.
  See also moral treatment
Cheney, Terri, 87, 88–89, 93
Child and Adolescent Bipolar
  Foundation, 121
Child and Adolescent Disorders Work
  Group, 120–121
children and bipolar disorder, 119–121
chlorpromazine, 112
chronic cases of insanity, 55–58
Chronic Diseases (Aretaeus of
  Cappadocia), 2–4
cingulated cortex, 103
circular insanity, 23–24
Clark, Michael, 118
classification systems: of asylum patients,
  45, 47, 51–54; Boerhaave's, 19; Bucknill
  and D. Tuke's, 24; in *DSM*, 26, 28–29;
  Esquirol's, 13–14, 21, 22; Falret's, 23;
  Kraepelin's, 24–25; Pinel's, 5, 20
class in asylums, 42–43, 51, 52–53
clinical efficacy of lithium, 113–114
Clinical Neuropharmacology Research
  Center, 101
Clinical Psychiatry (Kraepelin), 25
Cold Spring Harbor Laboratory, 66, 69
Commendium der Psychiatrie
  (Kraepelin), 25
communication revolution, 40
Comprehensive Textbook of Psychiatry
  (Freedman, Kaplan, and Sadock), 31–32,
  34–35
confinement to asylums, 48–51, 55
Conrad, Peter, 8
consensual reality, construction of,
  87–88
continuum, bipolar, 31, 32–34, 35
corpus callosum, 104
cortical atrophy, 102
corticolimbic network, 104
cortisol production, 103
criterion-based psychiatric diagnosis, 73
CT (computerized topographic) scans,
  101, 102
Cullen, William, 19

curability of insanity, 5, 41–42, 46,
    55–58, 67
custodial care, 56, 64

"dancing mania," 16, **17,** 18
Danvers State Insane Asylum, 59
Daston, Lorraine, 9
data resources for genomic research,
    78–79
Davenport, Charles, 69
deaths in asylums, 56–57
"democratic disease," 58
demonic attacks, 16
Department of Genetics for the Carnegie
    Institute, 69
depression as a neurosis, 30
*Description of the Retreat, an Institution
    near York, for Insane Persons of the
    Society of Friends* (S. Tuke), 37, 45
Detour (Simon), 84, 90
deviant behavior, mania as, 14
diagnosis: criterion-based psychiatric, 73;
    fear of in narratives, 92–93; molecular,
    79, 80; in narratives, 89–90, 91, 92–93;
    and patient interviews, 77
*Diagnostic and Statistical Manual of
    Mental Disorders (DSM),* 25, 26, 28–29;
    DSM-II, 30, 73; *DSM-IV,* 4; *DSM-IV-TR,*
    32–33; *DSM-V,* 119, 120–121
Dickens, Charles, 60, 61
DIGS ("Diagnostic Interview for Genetic
    Studies Self-Report"), 76–78
disease, multiple ontologies of, 7
distractibility, 25–26
Dix, Dorothea, 58, 59–60
double existence, 88. *See also* multiplicity
    of mania
drug therapies. *See* psychopharmaceuticals
Dryander, Johannes, **106**
*DSM. See Diagnostic and Statistical
    Manual of Mental Disorders*
Duganne, A.J.H., 61
Duke, Patty, 82
Dumit, Joseph, 105
Dunner, D. L., 32

Eastern Lunatic Asylum, 53, 56
Eggers, Dave, 82
ego, 30
Electroboy (Behrman), 81–82, 88
emotions, neuroimaging of, 101–103
epilepsy, 18
Esquirol, J.E.D. (Etienne), 5, 13–14, 20–21
"Esquirol's Patient, Part 1," **22**
eugenics movement, 66–70, **70, 71**
Eugenics Record Office, 66, 69

Falret, Jean Pierre, 23
family heredity studies, 11, 65, 70, 72–75.
    See also heredity
fear in mental illness narratives, 92–93
Fieve, Ronald R., 33
15q14 chromosomes, 76
*Finding Your Bipolar Muse: How to
    Master Depressive Droughts and Manic
    Floods and Access Your Creative Power*
    (Castle), 33
First Lines of the Practice of Physic
    (Cullen), 19
*First Report of the Physician of the
    Tennessee Lunatic Asylum: To the
    Legislature of Tennessee, for 1840 and
    1841,* 45–46
flashcards, eugenics, 69, **71**
fMRI scans, 101, 102, 110
Forkasdi, John, 86–87, 92, 93
"Forms of Insanity and Heredity of
    Patients" (*Iowa Medical Journal,*
    1895), 67
Foucault, Michel, 5–6, 39, 62, 63, 127n5,
    135n25
Freedman, Alfred M., 31
frenzy, 18
Freud, Sigmund, 30
Freudian psychoanalysis, 29–31
Friends Asylum at Frankford, 46
"Frier Hospital, London: a woman
    suffering from mania...", **109**
frontal lobe, degeneration of, 102
Frontline television program, 120
Fukuyama, Francis, 100
fury, 19–21, 24

Galen, 16, 19
Gartner, John D., 118–119
gaze, physician's, 39
genetics, 65–66, 70–76. *See also* eugenics
    movement; heredity
Genetics Initiative for Bipolar Disorder
    Consortium (Bipolar Consortium),
    75–76
"Genome-Wide Association of Bipolar
    Disorder in European American and
    African American Individuals"
    (*Molecular Psychiatry,* 2009), 76
genome-wide association studies, 79
genomic medicine, concerns of, 79
genomic research, 66, 75–79
gesture, Pinel's, 5, 40. *See also* chains,
    use of; moral treatment; Pinel,
    Philippe
Goshen, Charles, 15
grandiosity, 28, 87

Hacking, Ian, 7
hallucinations, 25
Hamilton, Linda, xi
Hare, Samuel, 55–56
Hawthorne, Nathaniel, 62
"Head and Brain of Adult Human Head,
    MRI," 107
Healy, David, 8, 112
hemoglobin, oxygenated, 102
heredity, 11, 64, 65, 67, 68, 69, 70, 70.
    See also eugenics movement; family
    heredity studies
Hermsen, Lisa: own experience with
    mania, 1–2, 10, 93–97, xii; participation
    in genetic study, 76–78
Hippocrates, 15, 19
Histories and Observations upon Most
    Diseases (Platter), 18
History of Madness (Foucault), 6, 39,
    135n25
Hollan, Holly, 86, 87, 89, 90, 92, 97
Hope, Melody, 89, 90, 92, 93
Hornbacher, Marya, 88, 89, 90–91, 92
Hospital for the Insane at Independence,
    Missouri, 67
House of Seven Gables (Hawthorne), 62
Huxley, Aldous, 100
hypersexuality, 87
hypomania, 31–32, 32–33, 118–119
Hypomanic Edge, The (Gartner), 118–119

iconography: of madness, 21; of mania, 2,
    3, 17–18, 27; of the maniac, 37–39, 39–41,
    107–110
Illinois State Hospital for the Insane, 54, 56
imaging technologies. See neuroimaging
    technologies
impulsivity, 87
inheritance as cause for mania, 64, 67
"Inherited Insanities" (Stewart), 68
In My Head (Hope), 89
Insane Asylum at Hartford, 60
Insane Asylum at South Boston, 60
insanity: asylums as only proper place for,
    46–47; categories of on admission
    records, 42; circular, 23–24; classes of, 51;
    as curable, 5, 41–42, 46, 55–58; heredity
    as cause of, 64, 67, 68; mania as worst
    class of, 40; quiet vs. violent, 50–51;
    theories for, 16; treatment for, 41–42.
    See also asylums; bipolar disorder; mania
In Small Doses (Pollard), 86
insomnia, 74, 103
International Neuropsychological
    Society, 2
interviews, patient, 72–73, 77

Iowa, eugenics in, 68–70
"Iowa 500 Study" (Winokur), 11, 65, 72–75
Iowa Medical Journal, 66–67
Iowa Psychopathic Hospital, 69
Iowa State Fair, 69

Jamison, Kay Redfield, 33, 96
Johnston, Suzy, 92–93
Journal of Insanity, 62–63

Kaplan, Harold I., 31, 34–35
Kean, Brian, 112, 135n25
Kern, Donald, 87, 89, 97
King, Larry, xi
Kirkbride, Thomas, 41, 43, 46–47, 54, 57–58
Kirkbride asylum model, 43
Klerman, G. L., 32
Kline, Nathan, 111
Knights of the Seal; or, the Mysteries of
    Three Cities: A Romance of Men's Hearts
    and Habits (Duganne), 61
Kraepelin, Emil, 10, 25–26, 27
Kramer, Peter, 112

Lakoff, Andrew, 116
Lamictal, 115
language: of brain functioning, 107; of
    madness, 33, 91–93; of mania, 19–21,
    103–104, xi; medicalized, 8, 88–90, 112; of
    mental illness, 83–84
Laughlin, Henry, 69
Law, John, 9
Let Them Eat Prozac (Healy), 112
Lily Pond, The (Barnes), 85, 88
limbic system, 104
Listening to Prozac (Kramer), 112
literature and fascination with maniacs,
    6, 62
lithium, 1, 90, 96, 110–115, 134n22. See also
    psychopharmaceuticals
Lunatic Asylum of South Carolina,
    45, 50, 53

madness: classes of, 51; classification of as
    inadequate system, 54; curability of, 5;
    description of, 6; iconography of, 21;
    language of, 33, 91–93; mania as, 4, 6;
    and mania in clinical descriptions,
    73–74; and mania in diagnostic
    interviews, 77; and mania in textbooks,
    14–15; in narrations, 83
"Madness" (Bell), 3
Madness (Hornbacher), 88
mania: as affective disorder, 34; author's
    experience with, 1–2, 10, 93–97, xii; as
    constructed, 124n3; cultural affinity for,

118–119; descriptions of, 2–4, 15–16, 19–21, 26, 30, 73–74; diagnostic criteria for in *DSM-IV-TR*, 28; in disciplinary publications, 8; Kraepelin concept of, 10, 26; as madness, 4, 19; in *New Oxford Textbook of Psychiatry*, 35; pathologization of, 31; pathophysiology of, 114; rhetorical history of, 2; role of clinical description and family history in diagnosing, 73–74; as specific madness, 6; as a state of mind, 20; in terms of regression, 31; theories of, 18, 19; as worst class of insanity, 40. *See also* asylums; bipolar disorder; insanity; madness; maniacs; narratives, mental illness; symptomology of mania

Mania and Depression: A Classification of Syndrome and Disease (Winokur), 64, 73

Mania: A Short History of Bipolar Disorder (Healy), 8

maniacs: asylum confinement of, 48–51, 55; description of, 15; iconic figure of, 2, 3, 37–39, 39–41; as icon of antebellum reform, 59; iconography of, 107–110; literary fascination with, 62; and public opinion, 40–41; as uncontrollable psychotic, 31

Manic: A Memoir (Cheney), 87

manic-depressive disorder. *See* bipolar disorder

Manic Depressive Insanity and Paranoia (Kraepelin), 25

"manic-depressive reactions," 26

manic episodes, 4, 34–35, 73–74

Manual of Psychological Medicine (Bucknill and D. Tuke), 23–24

markers, manic: genetic, 74–76; neuro, 101–104

marriage and insanity, 67

Martin, Emily, 9, 119

material consumption, anxiety and, 118

Maudsley, Henry, 129n61

medicalized language, 8, 88–90, 112

medical technologies. *See* neuroimaging technologies; psychopharmaceuticals

"Medicated Child, The" *(Frontline)*, 120

medication. *See* psychopharmaceuticals

melancholy, 18–19, 24

"Memoir on Circular Insanity" (Falret), 23

memoirs, mental illness. *See* narratives, mental illness

"Memorial to the Legislature of Massachusetts" (Dix), 59

memory as collective, 85–86

"mental hygiene," 117

mental illness. *See* bipolar disorder; insanity; madness; mania; narratives, mental illness

Mental Maladies: A Treatise on Insanity (Esquirol), 13–14

Metzl, Jonathan, 9

M'Gugin, D. L., 66–67

Middle Ages, mania in the, 16–18

Mind Gone Awry (Kern), 87

Mitchell, S. Weir, 117

mitochondrial DNA abnormalities, 74

Mol, Annemarie, 7, 9

"molecular diagnosis," 79, 80

molecular genetics, 75

monoamine oxidase inhibitors (MAOI), 110

mood disorders, neuroimaging of, 101–103

mood stabilizers, 110

moral treatment: and asylum architecture, 43; in asylum reform, 37; in asylum reports, 44–46; and drug-free alternatives, 111–112; and scientific objectivity, 135n25; S. Tuke's involvement with, 39; and violent patients, 52, 60. *See also* chains, use of

MRI (magnetic resolution imaging), 101, 102, 104, **107**, 110, 114

Müller-Wille, Staffan, 65

multiplicity of mania: in mental illness narratives, 84, 85, 88, 91–93; and the neuro future, 115–116; and neuroimaging, 104, 105, 110; in texts, 9–10

Mütter Museum of the College of Physicians, xi

Naked Birdwatcher, The (Johnston), 92–93

narratives, mental illness, 11, 81–97; and ability to narrate, 88–91; and bipolar collective, 85–86; fear of diagnosis in, 92–93; madness performed in, 83; mental illness as true debilitating condition in, 84–88; multiplicity of mania in, 91–93

National Alliance for Mental Illness, 119

National Human Genome Research Institute, 79

National Institute of Mental Health, 75, 101

National Institutes of Health, 79

Nazi eugenics program, 70

nerves, 16, 117

neurasthenia, 117

neuroimaging studies: bipolar as condition of, 104; on emotions, 102; on lithium, 114; and manic markers, 101–104; on mood disorders, 99, 101; multiplicity of, 104, 105

neuroimaging technologies, 11, 101–110; CT
scans, 101, 102; definitions of mania in
studies using, 103–104; ethical
consequences of, 99–100; importance of
difference in, 104–105; MRI/fMRI scans,
101, 102, 104, **107**, 110, 114; PET/SPECT,
101, 102–103, 110; promises of, 98; visual
rhetoric of, 105–107
neurological future, skeptics of, 99–100,
115–116
neuropsychological research, 35
neuropsychopharmaceuticals. *See*
psychopharmaceuticals
"Neuropsychopharmacology and the
Affective Disorders" (*New England
Journal of Medicine,* 1969), 114
neuroses, 30
new democracy in asylum reports, 46
New England Journal of Medicine, 114
New Hampshire Asylum, 52–53, 55
New Jersey State Lunatic Asylum, 53
New Oxford Textbook of Psychiatry, The
(Gelder, Andreasen, Lopez-Ibor, and
Geddes), 35
New York State Lunatic Asylum, 52, 53,
56–57
noises, 95

observations, importance of, 13
Observations on Maniacal Disorders
(Pargeter), 20
Ohio Lunatic Asylum, 42, 49, 55
ontologies of mania, multiple, 7
orbitofrontal cortex, 103, 104
Orr, Jackie, 9, 118
overdiagnosis: of bipolar disorder in
children, 120; of mental illness, 100

Palmer, Christopher, 87, 92, 93
*Panic Diaries: A Genealogy of Panic
Disorder* (Orr), 9, 118
panic disorder, 118
Paracelsus, 16–17
paralimbic seratonin 5-HT$_{1A}$ receptors,
101
Pargeter, William, 19–20
pathologization of social distress, 30–31
pathophysiology of mania, 114
patient interviews, 72–73
Pauley, Jane, 82
pedigree charts, 69, 70
Pennsylvania Hospital for the Insane,
41–42, 46–47, 54, 56, **57**, 57–58
PET (positron emission tomography), 101,
102–103
Pfizer company, 111

pharmacogenetics, 79. *See also*
psychopharmaceuticals
Pinel, Philippe, 5, 20, 37–39, **38**, 45–46, 61,
62. *See also* chains, use of; moral
treatment
Pinel, Scipion, 5
Platter, Felix, 18
Poe, Edgar Allen, 58, 60–61, 129n61
Politics of Life Itself, The (Rose), 98
Pollard, Marc, 86, 92
posthumanness, 115
prefrontal phosphomonoesters, 101
pressured speech, 25–26, 28, 89, 95–96
Prichard, Dr., 23–24
print culture, 44
privacy, neuroimaging and, 99–100
Prozac, 114
Prozac on the Couch (Metzl), 9
psychoanalysis, 29–32, 127n5
psychopathologies, 18
psychopharmaceuticals: critiques of, 100,
111–112; development technologies, 79,
98; discussion of in narratives, 90–91;
lithium, 1, 90, 96, 110–115, 134n22
psychosexuality, 30
psychosis, 12
public media: asylum rhetoric in, 58–62;
use of mania in, 119
public opinion: and asylum reports,
44–46, 51; and mania, 40–41

rage, 19–21, 24
rational treatment. *See* moral treatment
raving madness, 23–24
readmission of mania patients, 55–56
"recycled reality," 85–86
reform movements, 58. *See also* asylum
reform
regression, mania in terms of, 31
Reiss, Benjamin, 63
relapses, bipolar, 55–56, 119
*Report of the Board of Managers, for the
State of New York, A* (1880), 51
*Report of the Commissioners Appointed
by the Governor of New Jersey*
(1840), 49
*Report of the Officers of the Iowa Hospital
for the Insane* (1866), 51
*Report of the Pennsylvania Hospital for the
Insane for the Year 1883,* 57
*Report of the Superintendent of the Boston
Lunatic Hospital and Physician of the
Public Institution at South Boston*
(1840), 46
*Report of the Superintendent of the Lunatic
Asylum of South Carolina* (1842), 50

Report Relative to an Asylum for Lunatics, by the Joint Committee of Council and Assembly, Trenton (1841), 49–50
reports, asylum. *See* asylum reports
Reports of the Board of Visitors, of the Trustees, and of the Superintendent of the New Hampshire Asylum for the Insane (1843), 52–53
restraints. *See* chains, use of; moral treatment
Reynolds, David, 61
Rheinberger, Hans-Jörg, 65
rhetoric: Aristotelian, 6–7; asylum reform, 37–39, 58–62; visual, 105
rhetorical history of mania, 2
River Manic, The (Palmer), 87
Rose, Nikolas, 98, 116
Rush, Benjamin, 41

Sadock, Benjamin J., 31, 34–35
Sassi, Roberto B., 99
scans, brain. *See* brain scans; neuroimaging technologies
schizophrenia, 12
Schou, Morgen, 111
Scull, Andrew, 1
Secrets Within, The (Forkasdi), 86–87
Seroquel, 115
serotonin reuptake inhibitors (SRIs), 110
Shaffer, David, 121
Simon, Lizzie, 84, 85–86, 90, 92, 97
Singleton, Vickey, 9
Sixteenth Annual Report of the President and Directors of the Western Lunatic Asylum (1842), 52
slaves, insane, 53, 128n36
Smith-Kline and French company, 111
SNPs (single-nucleotide polymorphisms), 76, 79
Soares, Jair C., 99
Soaring and Crashing (Hollan), 86
social distress, pathologizing of, 30–31
Social Order/Mental Disorder (Scull), 1
social reform, asylums as symbolic of, 61
social status: and anxiety, 118; and classes of madness, 51, 52–53
SPECT (single-photon emission computed tomography), 101, 102–103, 110
speech, pressure of, 25–26, 28, 89, 95–96
spending, uncontrollable, 86–87, 94–95
State Asylum for New Jersey Lunatics, 55
state fairs, 69
Statistical Report of One Hundred and Ninety Cases of Insanity, Admitted into the Retreat near Leeds (Hare), 55–56
statistical tables, 42, 51, 67

Steadman, Keith Alan, 86, 90, 92
sterilization laws, 68–69. *See also* eugenics movement
Stewart, R. A., 68
St. John/St. Vitus dance, 16, 17, 18
storytelling, imaginative, 82
"Straitjacket" (Esquirol), 107, 108
suicidal behavior, 1, 94, 112, 119, 120
superego, 30
symbolic trauma, 30
symptomology of mania: distractibility, 25–26; evaluation of, 65, 72; fury, 19–21, 23–24; grandiosity, 28, 87; heightened activity, 34–35; hypersexuality, 87; impulsivity, 87; individual shape of in narratives, 86; insomnia, 74; noise sensitivity, 95; pressured speech, 25–26, 28, 89, 95–96; spending uncontrollably, 86–87, 94–95; suicidal behavior, 1, 94, 112, 119, 120
"System of Dr. Tarr and Professor Fether, The" (Poe), 60–61

technologies. *See* neuroimaging technologies; psychopharmaceuticals
temper dysregulation disorder with dysphoria, 120–121
textbooks, mania in, 14–15, 20, 23
Third Annual Report of the Directors of the Ohio Lunatic Asylum (1837), 49
Thompson, Charis, 9
Thompson, Jane, 89, 90, 92
Thurtle, Phillip, 70
toxicity of lithium, 113
treatment for insanity, 41–42. *See also* curability of insanity; moral treatment; psychopharmaceuticals
tricyclic antidepressants (TCA), 110
Tsuang, Ming T., 72
Tuke, Daniel H., 23–24
Tuke, Samuel, 37, 38, 39, 45, 46, 111, 135n25
Tuke, William, 39
Twenty-Fifth Annual Report of the Officers of the Vermont Asylum for the Insane, The (1861), 50
Twenty-Seventh Annual Report of the Officers of the Vermont Asylum for the Insane (1863), 50

United States, hypomania and, 118–119
University of Iowa Psychopathic Hospital, 65, 72
Unquiet Mind, The (Jamison), 96

Valium, 114
ventricular enlargement, 102

Vermont Asylum for the Insane, 50, 54
violent patients, 45, 50–51, 52, 53–54
visual rhetoric of neuroimaging
   technologies, 105

"wandering maniacs," 49
wealth and mania, 62–63
Western Lunatic Hospital, 52, 55
Whybrow, Peter C., 118

Willis, Thomas, 18–19
Winokur, George, 11, 64, 65, 72–75
Wirth-Couchan, Janet, 9
Woman and Borderline Personality
   (Wirth-Couchan), 9
Woodward, Samuel B., 46, 50
World Health Organization, 119

Zyprexa, 115

ABOUT THE AUTHOR

LISA M. HERMSEN is an associate professor and chair of the Department of English at the Rochester Institute of Technology, where she teaches courses in the rhetoric of science and the history of madness. *Manic Minds* was developed at the Philadelphia Library Company, where Hermsen received a fellowship from the Program in Early American Medicine, Science, and Society. While working on this manuscript, she served as the writing director at the Rochester Institute of Technology Institute. She has also published on gothic disability, presented on a research group using eye-tracking technology for composition practices, and written about the implications of teaching disciplinary writing conventions to deaf and hard-of-hearing student populations.

CPSIA information can be obtained at www.ICGtesting.com
Printed in the USA
BVOW070142071111

275441BV00001B/4/P